First Edition

Published by

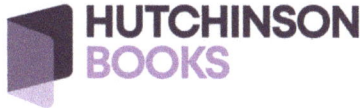

Spotting
the Signs

A Practical Guide to Red Flags for Clinicians

Introduction

In the fast-paced world of primary care and emergency medicine, the ability to recognise patterns and act decisively can mean the difference between timely intervention and missed opportunities. This book serves as a practical guide to aid in the early identification of red flags and differential diagnoses for common presentations in clinical practice.

Designed to be quick and accessible, this resource emphasises pattern recognition, guiding clinicians from initial symptoms to critical thinking and appropriate action. Each chapter is carefully structured, focusing on key features, red flags, and diagnostic frameworks such as the VITAMIN-C mnemonic. Our aim is to empower clinicians to navigate complex presentations with confidence, avoid pitfalls, and ensure optimal patient care.

Whether you're in the middle of a busy shift or revising for exams, this book is your go-to tool for concise, high-yield insights. We hope it provides clarity, support, and inspiration as you navigate the rewarding but demanding journey of medical practice.

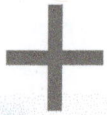

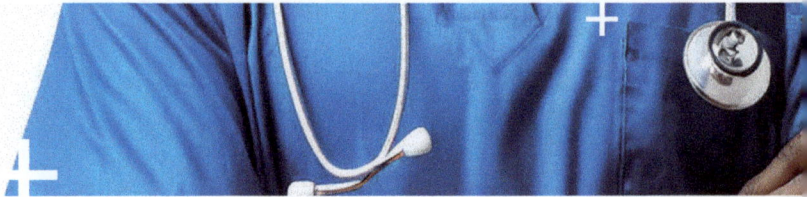
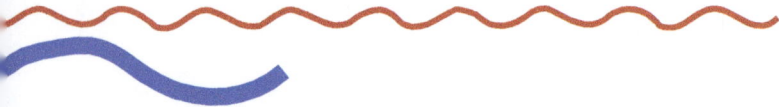
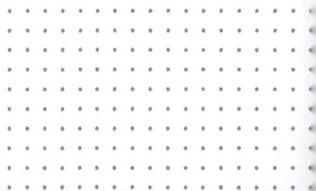

Spotting the Signs

A Practical Guide to Red Flags for Clinicians

Chapter		Page
01	Chest Pain	01
02	Syncope	11
03	Shortness of Breath	27
04	Cough	33
05	Haemoptysis	41
06	Hoarseness	49
07	Dyspepsia	55
08	Swollen Calf	65
09	Abdominal Pain	75
10	Constipation	81
11	Jaundice	87
12	Diarrhoea	97
13	Vomiting	105
14	Haematemesis	113
15	Rectal Bleeding	121
16	Dysphagia	126
17	Haematuria	135
18	Headache	141
19	Dizziness	149
20	Vertigo	155
21	Double Vision	161
22	Sudden Vision Loss	169
23	Ataxia	177
24	Tremor	185
25	Numbness and paraesthesia	193
26	Seizure	201
27	Back pain	209
28	Rash	217

Written by Dr. Zaira Jawaid Akhtar, Dr. Torti Obasi
Co-authors Dr. Alexander Sherlock, Dr. Shezal Hussain
Corresponding Author Dr. Amir Ahmad

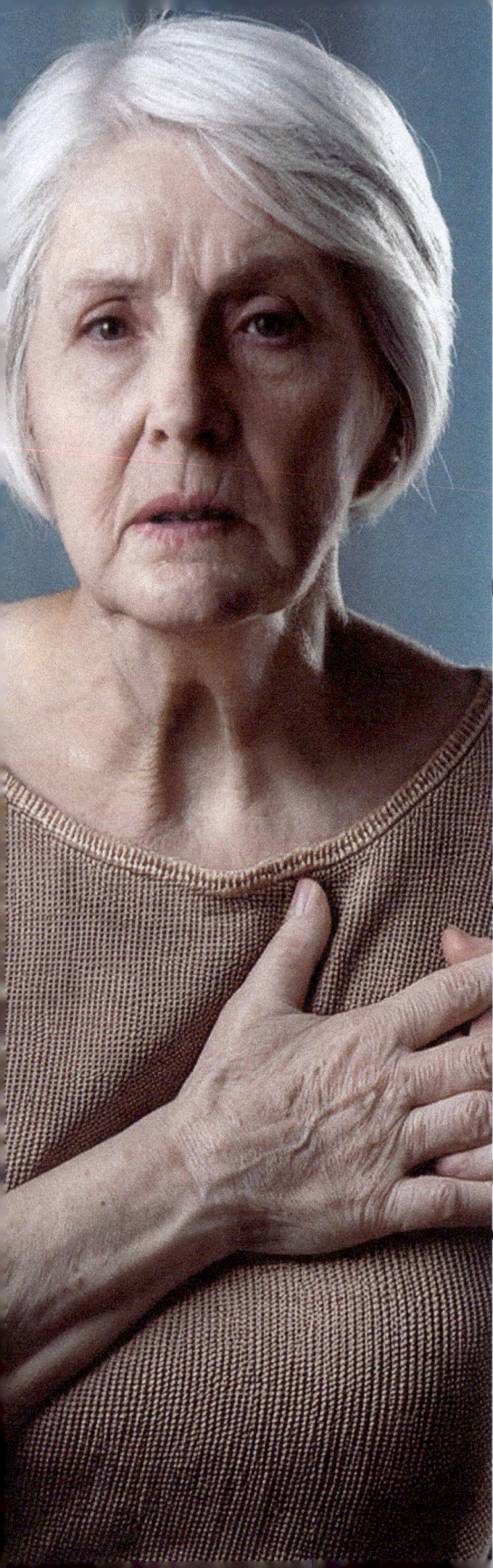

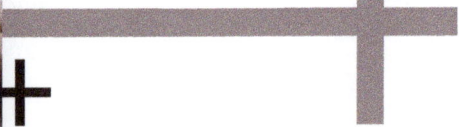

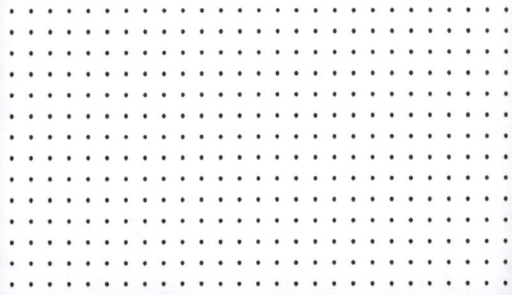

01
Chest Pain

Chest pain is one of the most frequent yet critical symptoms in clinical practice. It results from myriad causes, from benign conditions like musculoskeletal strain to life-threatening emergencies such as myocardial infarction, pulmonary embolism, and aortic dissection. Accurate and prompt evaluation is essential to differentiate between these causes and prioritize high-risk conditions. A systematic approach and recognizing red flags helps narrow the differential diagnosis and ensures timely intervention.

Diagnostic sieves

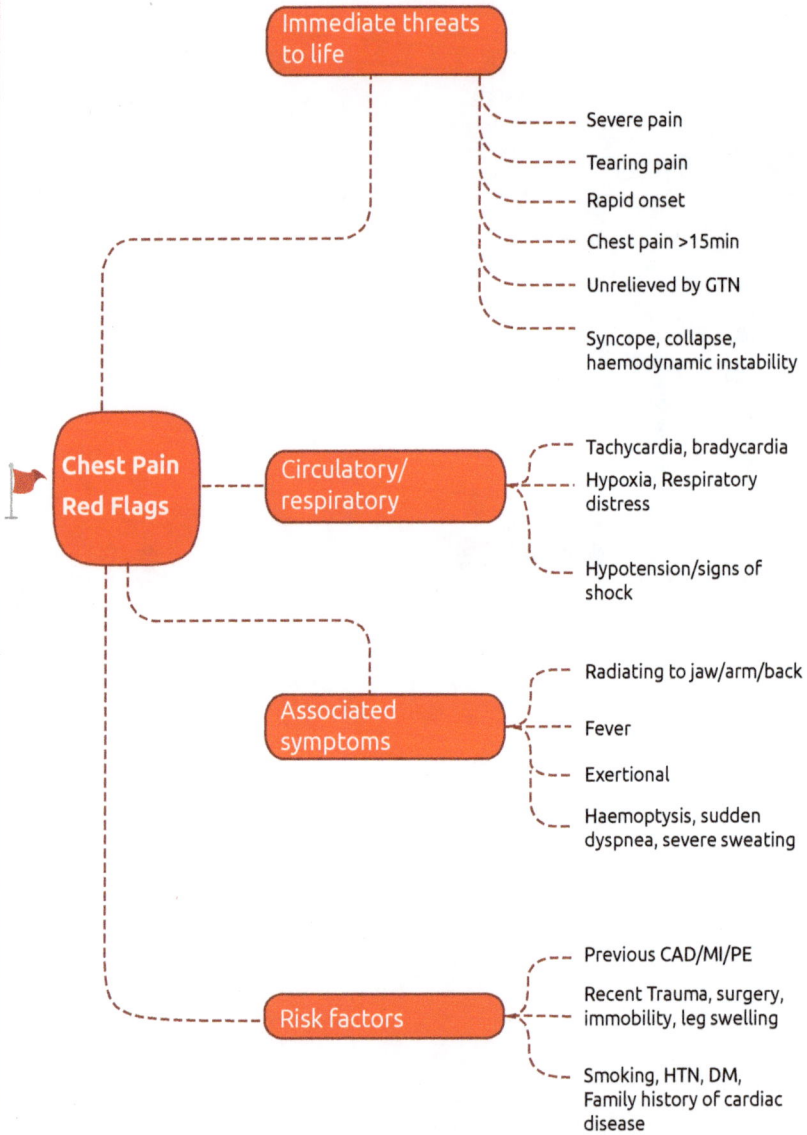

Chest Pain Red Flags

Immediate threats to life
- Severe pain
- Tearing pain
- Rapid onset
- Chest pain >15min
- Unrelieved by GTN
- Syncope, collapse, haemodynamic instability

Circulatory/respiratory
- Tachycardia, bradycardia
- Hypoxia, Respiratory distress
- Hypotension/signs of shock

Associated symptoms
- Radiating to jaw/arm/back
- Fever
- Exertional
- Haemoptysis, sudden dyspnea, severe sweating

Risk factors
- Previous CAD/MI/PE
- Recent Trauma, surgery, immobility, leg swelling
- Smoking, HTN, DM, Family history of cardiac disease

History Taking

ONSET:

- Sudden, severe pain is concerning for MI, PE, aortic dissection, or pneumothorax.
- Gradual onset suggests GERD, musculoskeletal pain, or pericarditis.

CHARACTER:

- Crushing or heavy: Indicative of MI.
- Tearing or ripping: Aortic dissection.
- Burning or retrosternal: GERD or oesophageal issues.
- Sharp and pleuritic: PE, pneumothorax, or pericarditis.

RADIATION:

- Pain to the jaw, arms, or neck suggests cardiac origin
- To the back indicates aortic dissection or oesophageal issues.

ASSOCIATED SYMPTOMS:

- Sweating, nausea: MI.
- Breathlessness: PE, pneumothorax, pneumonia.
- Fever: Pericarditis, pneumonia.
- Haemoptysis: PE or malignancy.

EXERTION AND POSITIONING:

- Exertional chest pain relieved by rest: Likely angina or MI.
- Pain relieved leaning forward: Pericarditis.
- Pain worse after eating: GERD.

RISK FACTORS:

- For MI: Hypertension, smoking, diabetes, family history.
- For PE: Recent immobility, surgery, pregnancy, malignancy.
- For pneumothorax: COPD, trauma, young tall males.
- For malignancy: smoker, weight loss, asbestos exposure, chronic cough, intractable chest wall pain.
- For oesophageal rupture: recent endoscopy, copious vomiting or retching

Differential diagnoses of chest pain sorted with the VITAMIN-C framework

Category	Differential Diagnosis
Vascular	Myocardial infarction (MI), Pulmonary embolism (PE), Aortic dissection
Infectious	Pneumonia, Pericarditis, Mediastinitis
Trauma	Rib fractures, Pneumothorax, Oesophageal rupture
Autoimmune	Systemic lupus erythematosus (SLE), Rheumatoid arthritis
Metabolic	Hyperthyroidism, Anaemia
Idiopathic/Functional	Panic attacks, Anxiety
Neoplastic	Lung cancer, Mesothelioma, Oesophageal carcinoma
Degenerative	Intercostal neuralgia, Musculoskeletal pain
Congenital	Marfan syndrome

Diagnostic sieves
■ □ □ □ +

Serious diagnoses to consider

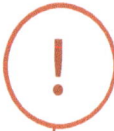

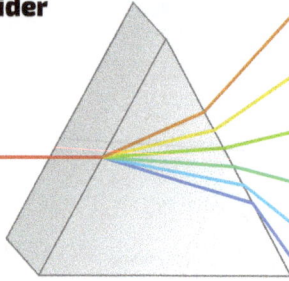

(!)

- Myocardial Infarction
- Pulmonary Embolism
- Aortic Dissection
- Pneumothorax
- Pericarditis and/or Cardiac Tamponade
- Oesophageal Rupture

(!) SERIOUS SYMPTOMS!

- Central chest pain radiating to arm, jaw, or neck: Suggestive of **cardiac ischemia**, especially if associated with sweating or nausea.
- Tearing or ripping pain radiating to the back: Strongly indicates **aortic dissection.**
- Sharp, pleuritic pain aggravated by deep breaths: Seen in **PE, pneumothorax, or pleuritis.**
- Burning or retrosternal pain post-meals: Suggests **GERD or oesophageal issues.**
- Pain relieved by leaning forward: Often seen in **pericarditis.**
- Sudden, unilateral chest pain with dyspnoea: Suggestive of **pneumothorax.**
- Severe pain following vomiting or retching: Indicates **oesophageal rupture.**

(!) SERIOUS SIGNS!

- Elevated troponins and ECG changes (e.g., ST elevation): Point to **myocardial infarction.**
- Hypoxemia, tachycardia, and D-dimer elevation: Suggest **pulmonary embolism.**
- Widened mediastinum on imaging: Seen in **aortic dissection.**
- Decreased or absent breath sounds: Indicative of **pneumothorax.**
- Pericardial rub on auscultation: Typical of **pericarditis.**
- Subcutaneous emphysema or mediastinal air: Found in o**esophageal rupture.**
- Beck's triad (muffled heart sounds, raised JVP, and hypotension): Points to **cardiac tamponade.**

Serious diagnoses to consider

I. MYOCARDIAL INFARCTION (MI)

Pain from myocardial ischemia and oesophageal reflux can mimic each other, sharing a burning nature and radiating to similar areas like the back or arms.

ECG changes strongly suggest MI, though a normal ECG does not exclude unstable angina. Troponin testing is critical for ruling out MI.

Cardiac risk factors may warrant further evaluation with an exercise tolerance test (ETT) or echocardiography if the diagnosis is uncertain.

2. AORTIC DISSECTION

Often presents with sudden, severe, tearing pain radiating to the back.

Risk factors include Marfan's syndrome, bicuspid aortic valve, and blood pressure or pulse deficits.

Associated symptoms may include neurological deficits (e.g., hemiparesis, paraparesis), haematuria, and abdominal or lower back pain.

Clinical diagnosis is supported by a widened mediastinum on CXR or the presence of clinical signs like pulse deficits (positive likelihood ratio +10).

3. TENSION PNEUMOTHORAX

A medical emergency presenting with severe dyspnoea, tachycardia, hypotension, and signs like distended neck veins and tracheal deviation.

Auscultation reveals reduced air entry on the affected side; no time for a confirmatory chest X-ray.

Features on imaging (when obtained) include contralateral mediastinal shift, hyper-expanded hemithorax, and depressed hemidiaphragm.

Are you missing something?

- Always consider **aortic dissection** in patients with tearing chest pain and pulse discrepancies.
- Suspect **PE** in pleuritic pain with risk factors for venous thromboembolism.
- **Oesophageal rupture** requires urgent diagnosis if pain follows vomiting or retching.

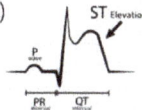

EMNote

ST Elevation - Not Always AMI

Mnemonic for causes of ST elevation : "ELEVATION"

E : Electrolytes (e.g. hyperkalemia)
L : Left bundle branch block
E : (Benign) Early repolarization
V : Ventricular hypertrophy
A : Arrhythmia (Brugada, VT), Aneurysm of LV, Aortic dissection
T : Takotsubo disease, Traumatic brain injury (ICH)
I : Infarct (MI), Injury(contusion), Inflammation (myo/peri-carditis)
O : Osborn (J) waves (hypothermia or hypercalcemia)
N : Non-atherosclerotic vasospasm (Prinzmetal's angina)

@ jackcfchong

Top Tips

PLEURITIC CHEST PAIN

The initial probabilities for causes of pleuritic chest pain when presenting in an emergency department vary significantly, depending on the underlying condition:

- **Musculoskeletal causes:** Approximately 45% of cases. This is the most common cause and includes costochondritis and other chest wall pain.
- **Chest infections:** Around 22%, which may include pneumonia and bronchitis, often accompanied by fever and productive cough.
- **Pneumothorax:** Accounts for 7% of cases, typically presenting with acute onset dyspnoea and reduced breath sounds.
- **Pleurisy (non-infective causes):** 6%, which can result from inflammation of the pleura due to autoimmune conditions or other causes.
- **Pulmonary embolism (PE):** Incidence ranges from 1% to 21%, depending on clinical presentation and risk factors, such as recent surgery, immobility, or malignancy.
- **Acute pericarditis:** Less than 1%, presenting with positional chest pain and possibly a pericardial friction rub

CLINICAL PATTERNS AND RED FLAGS

- Persistent chest pain >15 minutes, especially with sweating or nausea, is highly suggestive of cardiac origin.
- A normal ECG does not exclude MI; serial testing is essential.
- Tearing pain radiating to the back and unequal pulses is pathognomonic for aortic dissection.

APPROACH AND RISK STRATIFICATION

- TIMI score or HEART score can help stratify risk in suspected ACS.
- Wells score can aid in assessing the likelihood of PE.
- CT angiography is critical for suspected aortic dissection or PE.

Important ECG patterns

STEMI & STEMI EQUIVALENTS:

These patterns often indicate acute myocardial infarction requiring urgent reperfusion therapy.

1. Lateral Wall STEMI

- ST-elevation in lateral leads (I, aVL, V5, V6).
- Reciprocal ST-depression in inferior leads (III, aVF).
- High Lateral STEMI: ST-elevation primarily in leads I and aVL.
- Clinical Note: Prompt recognition ensures timely PCI activation.

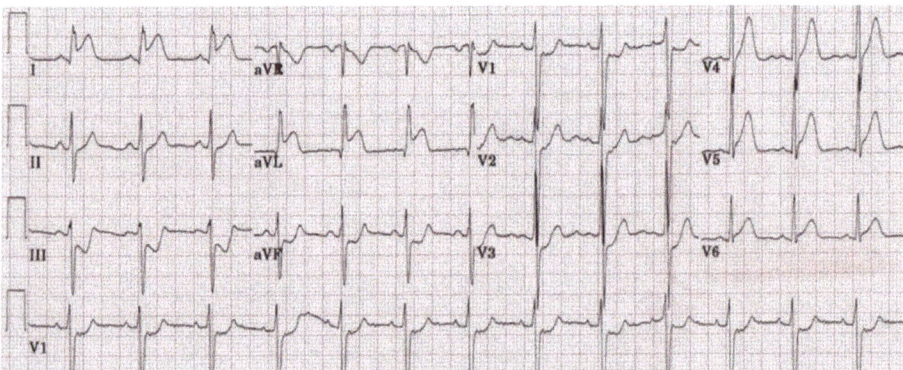

Figure 4.1: High Lateral STEMI; *litfl.com/lateral-stemi-ecg-library*

2. De Winter's T Waves

Significance: Proximal LAD occlusion (seen in ~2% of patients).

ECG Features:

*   Up-sloping ST-depression at the J-point in V1–V4 (without STE).
*   Tall, symmetric T-waves in V1–V4.
*   Possible ST-elevation in aVR and/or aVL

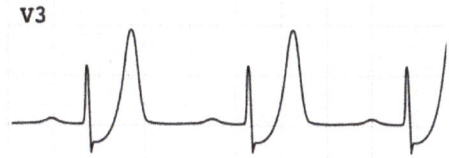
Figure 4.2: De Winter T Waves: Upsloping ST depression and peaked T waves in precordial leads; *litfl.com/de-winter-t-wave*

3. Left Main Coronary Artery Stenosis

*   ST-elevation in aVR and/or aVL.
*   Widespread ST-depression in leads I, II, and V4–V6.
*   Often associated with cardiogenic shock if complete occlusion is present.

4. Posterior Wall MI

*   ST-depression and upright T-waves in V1–V3.
*   Horizontal ST-depression in these leads with prominent R-waves.
*   Confirm with posterior leads (V7–V9) showing ST-elevation.

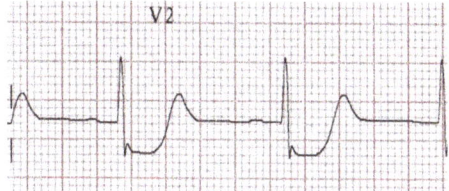
Figure 4.3: Posterior infarction in V2; litfl.com/posterior-myocardial-infarction-ecg-library

5. Wellen's Syndrome

Significance: Critical LAD stenosis.

ECG Findings:

*   Deeply inverted or biphasic T waves in V2–V3 (may extend to V1–V6).

Normal troponins do not rule out Wellen's syndrome.

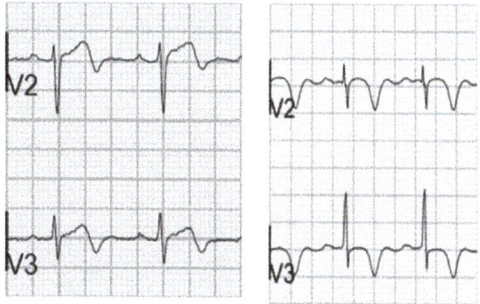
Wellens pattern A: Biphasic T waves

Wellens pattern B: Deeply inverted T waves

Figure 4.4: Wellens
emra.org/students/newsletter-articles/wellens-and-brugada

NON-STEMI CAUSES OF ST ELEVATION

These conditions may mimic STEMI but require different management strategies.

Benign Early Repolarization (BER)

*   Early repolarization is a common and benign ECG finding, particularly in young, healthy individuals.
*   It presents as diffuse ST-segment elevation, most prominent in the precordial leads, characterized by an elevated J-point, often referred to as a "high take-off."
*   The ST elevation typically has a concave shape.

ECG:

*   Concave upward ST-elevation with distinct J-point notching.
*   Diffuse distribution, often most pronounced in V3–V4.
*   No reciprocal changes or evolving patterns.

Left Bundle Branch Block (LBBB)

*   Wide, negative QS complex in V1.
*   Tall, broad R-waves in V6.
*   STE in V1–V3.

Appropriate Discordance:

- Opposite deflection of QRS and ST segments (e.g., ST-elevation with a negative QRS).
- In normal LBBB wherever the QRS is up ST is down (e.g lead V1, V2) and wherever the QRS is down the ST is up. This is called appropriate discordance. If both are in the same direction (QRS is up and ST is up), this is called inappropriate concordance and is suggestive of STEMI. It is highly specific but not sensitive (found in some patients only).

Left Ventricular Hypertrophy (LVH)

- High-voltage R-waves in lateral leads and deep S-waves in anterior leads.

- Possible STE in V1–V3.

Takotsubo Cardiomyopathy

- Often mimics anterior STEMI with ST-elevation but typically resolves without coronary artery occlusion.

Traumatic Brain Injury

- Can present with diffuse ST elevation

Pulmonary Embolism

- Can cause ST segment elevation with RBBB

Key Differentiation Strategies

I. STEMI VS. PERICARDITIS

- Is there ST-depression in leads other than aVR or V1? If yes, STEMI.
- Is the ST-elevation convex or horizontal? If yes, STEMI.
- Is ST-elevation in lead III greater than in lead I? If yes, STEMI.

- If the answer is No to ALL of the above questions, then look for PR segment depression in multiple leads. PR segment depression is not specific for Pericarditis and can also happen in STEMI.

Pericarditis: Concave ST-elevation with PR depression, no reciprocal changes.

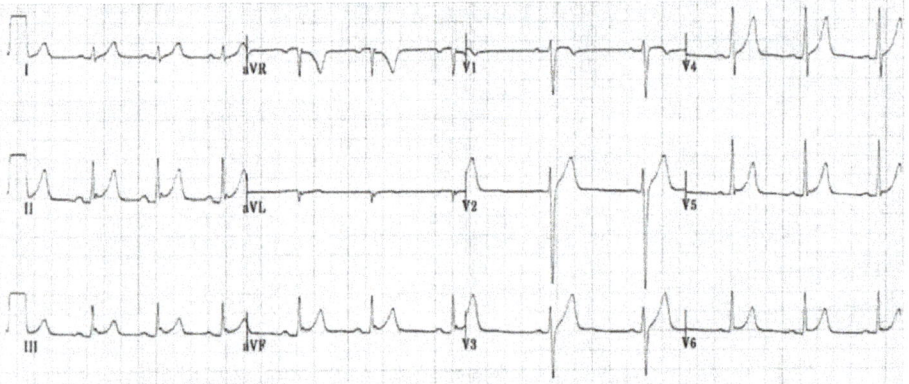

Figure 4.5: (Above) BER;
litfl.com/benign-early-repolarisation-ecg-library

Figure 4.6: (Left) LBBB; Dominant S wave in V1, Broad and notched R wave in V6
litfl.com/left-bundle-branch-block-lbbb-ecg-library

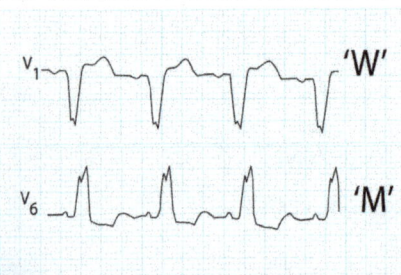

2. STEMI VS. BENIGN EARLY REPOLARISATION (BER)

Although considered harmless, distinguishing early repolarization from pathological ST elevation, such as that seen in acute myocardial infarction or pericarditis, can be challenging.

Misinterpretation may lead to missed diagnoses of STEMI or unnecessary interventions for non-STEMI cases.

BER is diffuse, without reciprocal changes, and has stable characteristics across serial ECGs.

STEMI often shows reciprocal ST-depression, poor R-wave progression, and evolving changes.

ECG characteristics that are more likely to be seen in BER include:

- ST elevation at the J-point with upward concavity ("smiley" face)
- Notching of the J-point
- Diffuse ST elevation (typically highest in V3-4)
- Concordant, prominent T-waves with large amplitudes
- Normal R-wave progression
- Relative stability from one ECG to the next

Further tips:

- Avoid relying solely on ST-segment morphology to exclude acute myocardial infarction (AMI), as approximately 40% of anterior myocardial infarctions present with up-sloping (concave) ST-segment elevation.
- Exercise caution when diagnosing benign early repolarization (BER) if there is poor R-wave progression, anterior Q-waves, inferior ST depression, or terminal QRS distortion.
- Be particularly wary of diagnosing BER in patients over 55 years old or those with concerning clinical symptoms.
- When subtle STEMI is a concern, use additional tools such as serial ECGs, comparison with prior ECGs for further evaluation.

3. STEMI VS. LV ANEURYSM

Persistent, coved ST-elevation with Q-waves in anterior leads suggests LV aneurysm rather than acute STEMI.

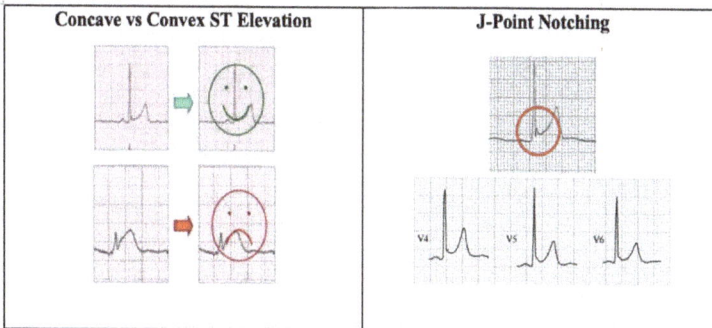

Figure 4.7: Difference in morphology between BER ("smiley" face) and STEMI ("frowny" face), and J-point notching seen in BER
emnote.org/emnotes/causes-of-st-elevation-in-ecg

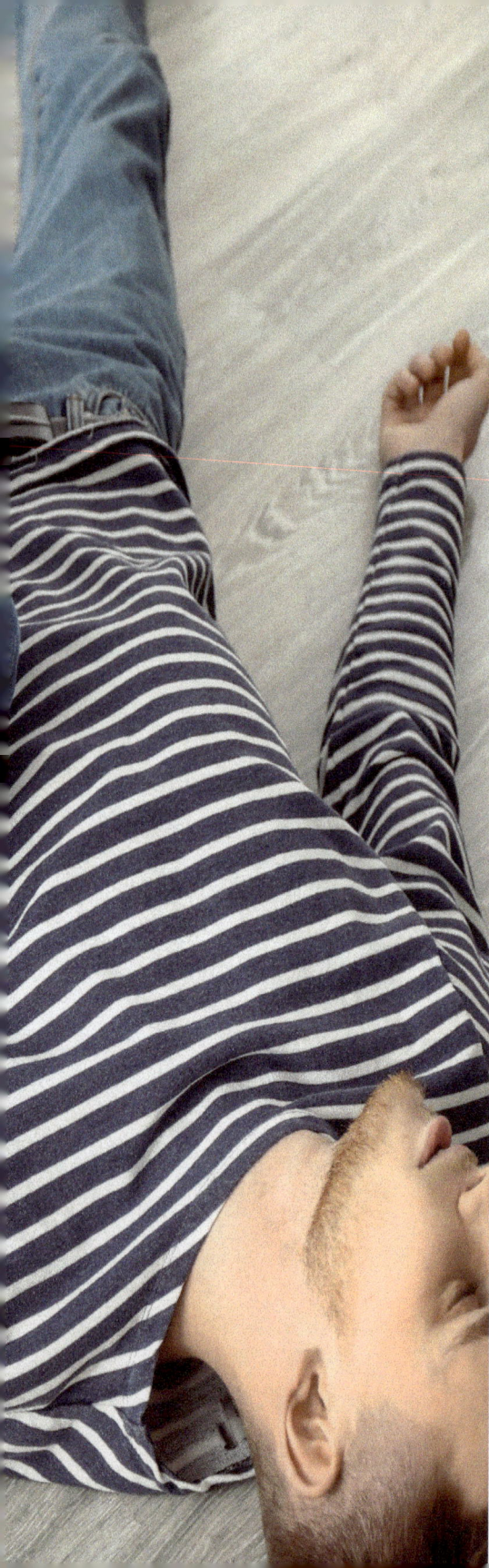

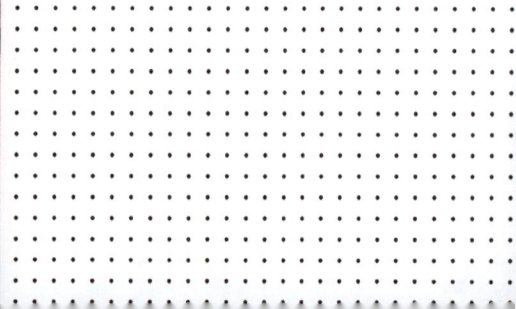

02
Syncope

The commonest cause of transient loss of consciousness, **syncope** is due to cerebral hypoperfusion and is a common yet complex presentation in the emergency room with key implications for accurate diagnosis and management because it can be a sign of both benign conditions and life-threatening illnesses. This chapter offers tools to demistify and simplying approaching patient presenting with syncope.

Syncope Red Flags

- **Cardiac/circulatory**
  - *Abnormal ECG findings
  - Exertional syncope
  - Family history of sudden cardiac death; OR personal history of heart disease
  - Associated palpitations
  - Associated chest pain or dyspnoea
  - Hypotension
  - Persistent bradycardia
  - Cardiac murmur
  - **Syncope when supine; syncope when seated/driving

- **Non cardiac/neurological**
  - GI/rectal bleed
  - Anaemia
  - Hypoglycemia,
  - Dyselectrolytaemia

- **Neurological**
  - Absence of or short (<10s) prodrome
  - Prolonged confusion
  - Focal neurological deficits
  - Preceding Trauma

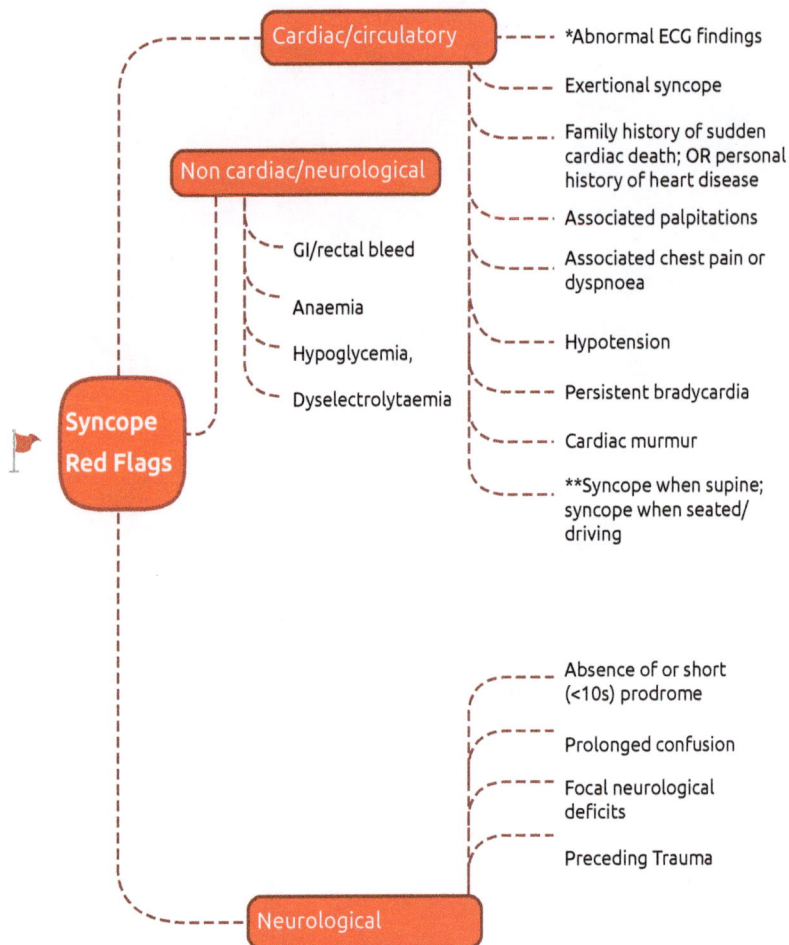

*Abnormal ECG findings ie. Mobitz 2nd degree or 3rd degree heart block, pre-excitation (wolf-parkinson-white, Lown-Ganong-Levine), Long/short QT interval, Ischemic changes etc.
**Syncope when supine - sleep vasovagal syncope, epilepsy

History Taking

ONSET:

- When did the event occur - time of day?
- Onset sudden vs gradual?
- Were they standing, sitting, or lying down?
- Any emotional triggers (e.g., fear, pain, or stress)?
- Was there a warning?
- Symptoms like lightheadedness, dizziness, nausea, or sweating (suggests vasovagal syncope).
- Palpitations preceding the event (suggests arrhythmia). Complete absence of warning (suggests arrhythmias or seizure).

CHARACTER:

Describe the event:

- Was there complete loss of consciousness and postural tone? How long?
- Any associated convulsive movements, tongue biiting, eye rolling, incontinence? (suggests seizure)

Recovery:

- Rapid with no confusion (suggests vasovagal syncope)
- Prolonged confusion or fatigue (suggests seizure)

ASSOCIATED SYMPTOMS:

Symptoms before or during the event:

- Chest pain or discomfort radiating to the arm/jaw, or back (suggests ischemic heart disease or aortic dissection)
- Dyspnea or chest tightness (suggests pulmonary embolism or heart failure)
- Neck pain or headache (suggests carotid artery dissection or raised intracranial pressure)
- Palpitations? (suggests arrhythmia)
- Focal weakness, vision changes, or speech disturbances (suggests stroke or TIA)
- Headache or neck stiffness (suggests raised intracranial pressure or meningitis)
- Fever, night sweats, or unexplained weight loss (suggests infection or malignancy)
- Dark urine or pale stools (suggests liver dysfunction or hemolysis)
- Breathlessness or hemoptysis (suggests pulmonary embolism)
- Symptoms of hypoglycemia such as sweating or shakiness.
- Actions like lip-smacking, a rising feeling in the stomach, experiencing déjà vu, convulsive movements or incontinence (suggest a seizure)

EXERTION AND POSITIONING:

Exertion:

- Did the syncope occur during exertion or immediately afterward? (suggests cardiac causes such as hypertrophic cardiomyopathy or arrhythmias)

Positioning:

- Did the event occur while/after prolonged standing, sitting, or lying down?
- Were symptoms triggered by prolonged standing or relieved by lying down (suggests orthostatic hypotension or vasovagal syncope)?

RISK FACTORS:

Cardiac Causes:

- Family history of sudden cardiac death (<40 years)
- Personal history of heart failure, arrhythmias, or structural heart disease.
- Use of medications that prolong the QT interval.

Neurological Causes:

- History of seizures or other neurological disorders (e.g., epilepsy, TIA).
- Head trauma associated with the event.

Orthostatic Hypotension:

- Recent surgery, dehydration, or prolonged immobility.
- Use of antihypertensive medications or diuretics.
- Dysautonomia: History of Parkinsons disease, diabetes

Pulmonary Embolism (PE):

- Recent immobilization, surgery,

Serious diagnoses to consider

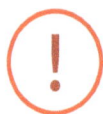

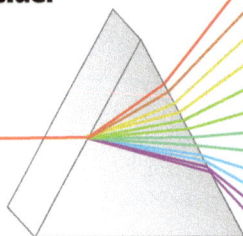

Arrhythmias (Stokes Adams Attack, Ventricular tachycardia)

Complete Heart Block

Hypertrophic Cardiomyopathy

Aortic Stenosis

Myocardial Infarction

Aortic Dissection

Pulmonary Embolism

Status Epilepticus

Stroke/TIA

Carotid Artery Dissection/ Stenosis

Haemorrhage (including SAH)

Metabolic (Hypoglycaemia, Adrenal Insufficiency, Acute Intoxication or Poisoning)

! SERIOUS SYMPTOMS!

- Palpitations before syncope; chest pain or pressure; breathlessness or dyspnea. Think **cardiac arrhythmias, ischeamia, PE.**
- Sudden-onset headache; focal neurological deficits (e.g., weakness, vision changes); confusion or prolonged post-event disorientation. Think **neurologic** causes
- Sudden fatigue or dizziness; severe abdominal or back pain; dark or tarry stools (indicating GI bleeding). Think systemic causes - **hypoxia, hypoglycaemia, anaemia**
- Recent trauma or head injury; severe nausea or vomiting before the event. These suggest **intracranial SOL/ haematoma**

! SERIOUS SIGNS!

- ECG Conduction abnormalities (e.g., heart block, sick sinus, prolonged QT, ischaemic ST-segment changes)
- Systolic BP <90mmHg; persistent bradycardia <40 bpm or tachycardia >120bpm; suggestive of **shock, adrenal insufficiency, medication or arrhythmia**
- Focal neurological deficits (e.g., **hemiparesis, dysarthria**) suggests stroke. Neck stiffness (suggesting **meningitis or subarachnoid hemorrhage**). Signs of raised intracranial pressure (e.g., papilledema on fundoscopy) suggest **intracranial bleed/lesion.**
- Pallor, tachycardia suggest **anaemia.** Jaundice (suggesting **liver failure**). Cyanosis (suggesting **hypoxia or pulmonary embolism**).

Differential diagnoses of Syncope using VITAMIN CDE acronym

Several causes from the VITAMIN CDE framework are attributable to orthostatic hypotension, either directly or indirectly through mechanisms like autonomic dysfunction, hypovolemia, or impaired vascular tone; this framework is recommended here solely as a mnemonic device.

V	VASCULAR	**Orthostatic Hypotension** Primary Autonomic failure	Parkinson's disease
			Multiple System Atrophy
			Pure autonomic failure (rare)
			Lewy Body Dementia
		Orthostatic Hypotension Secondary Autonomic failure	Diabetes mellitus (autonomic neuropathy)
			Chronic kidney disease
			Spinal cord injuries
			Amyloidosis
			Alcohol-induced neuropathy
			Fever
			Dehydration (vascular insufficiency)
		Dysautonomias	Postural Orthostatic Tachycardia Syndrome (POTS)
			Carotid sinus syndrome
			Neurocardiogenic syncope
		Structural	Aortic dissection (rare)
			Subclavian steal syndrome (rare)
			Takayasu arteritis (rare)
I	INFECTIOUS	**Severe Infections**	Septic shock.
			Myocarditis
		Neurological Infections Others	Neurocysticercosis (in endemic regions; rare)
			Meningitis
T	TOXICOLOGICAL	**Medications:**	Tricyclic antidepressants
			Beta-blockers
			Organophosphates (rare)
		Others	Alcohol or drug intoxication
			Carbon monoxide poisoning
A	AUTOIMMUNE		Systemic lupus erythematosus (SLE)
			Sarcoidosis (rare)
			Autoimmune autonomic neuropathy (rare)
M	METABOLIC	**Electrolyte Imbalances**	Hypokalemia
			Hyperkalemia
		Others	Severe anemia
			Haemorrhage
I	IDIOPATHIC		Vasovagal syncope
			Situational syncope (triggers: cough, swallowing, urination)
N	NEUROLOGICAL	**Seizures**	Seizures/Epilepsy
		Cerebrovascular Events	Stroke
			Transient ischemic attack
			Subarachnoid hemorrhage
			Carotid artery dissection (rare)
C	CARDIAC	**Arrhythmias**	Ventricular tachycardia
			Complete heart block
			Long QT syndrome
		Structural	Hypertrophic cardiomyopathy
			Aortic stenosis
			Cardiac tamponade (rare)
		Ischaemic	Myocardial infarction
D	DEGENERATIVE		Parkinson's disease (with autonomic involvement)
			Multiple System Atrophy (MSA)
E	ENVIRONMENTAL		Heat stroke
			High-altitude cerebral oedema (HACE) **(rare)**
			Acute hypoxia due to environmental factors (e.g., carbon monoxide)

malignancy, or history of thrombophilia.

Metabolic Causes:

- Hypoglycemia (e.g., diabetes, missed meals).
- Thyrotoxicosis or adrenal insufficiency.

Vasovagal Syncope:

- Triggers like emotional distress, pain, or prolonged standing.
- Symptoms in crowded or hot environments.

HELPFUL HISTORY-TAKING TIPS

Is this true syncope or something else (eg, stroke, seizure, head injury)?

Mnemonic to recall specific questions to ask, expands on the 3 Ps concepts:

5 Ps - **Precipitant, Prodrome, Position, Palpitations, Post-event phenomena**

5 Cs - **Colour, Convulsions, Continence, Cardiac Problems, Cardiac Death Family history**

↓

If this is true syncope, is there a clear life-threatening cause?

Risk factors for serious cause:

- Exertion preceding the event
- Note that syncope during exertion much more concerning than syncope after exertion
- No preceding symptoms
- Concerning for cardiac dysrhythmia
- History of cardiac disease in the patient
- Family history of sudden death, or cardiac disease
- Recurrent episodes
- Recumbent episode
- Prolonged loss of consciousness
- Associated chest pain, shortness of breath or palpitations

↓

If this is true syncope and the cause is not clear, is the patient at high risk for serious outcome?

Run through serious causes:

Cardiovascular-mediated syncope
- Usually absence of prodrome

History of structural heart disease
- Family history of sudden cardiac death
- Syncope during exertion

Chest pain or palpitations associated with syncope
- Abnormal ECG

Neurally mediated syncope
- Trigger event (fear/pain/prolonged standing/warm environment)
- Prodrome of nausea/vomiting, tunnel vision, lightheadedness, diaphoresis, warmth
- Associated with head movement or pressure on neck: commonly occurs while shaving, when in church/wearing a tight collar.

Orthostatic hypotension-mediated syncope
- After standing up
- Change in medications

WHEN TO ADMIT

San Francisco Syncope Rule (SFSR) was designed to have 96% Sensitivity for identifying patients at immediate risk for serious outcome with 7 days.

The Mnemonic for feature of the rule is **"CHESS"**

C   - h/o CCF

H   - Haematocrit < 30 %

E   - ECG abnormalities

S   - Shortness of breath

S   - Triage systolic BP < 90

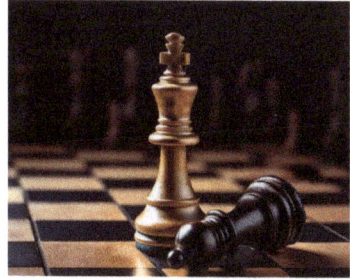

A patient with any of the above is considered at high risk for a serious outcome such as death MI, PE, Stroke, SAH, signifier haemorrhage or any condition causing a return to ED and hospitalisation for a related event.

As recommended by the authors the rule should be used during the initial evaluation of syncope at the discretion of the ED Physician treating the patient and should include all available ECGs and results of cardiac monitoring . In patients without an evident cause of syncope and a negative San Francisco rule the result of serious outcome is 2% allowing for safe discharge.

A patient meeting the SFSR criteria will have a 10% risk of serious outcome (such as death, myocardial infarction, pulmonary embolism, stroke, or another significant event) and 0.4% risk of sudden death. The incident of sudden death is high after the onset of symptoms which are usually exertional in nature.

Summary of concepts so far:

See if you can keep a systematic approach to ensure all potential causes are considered and appropriately investigated:

1. INITIAL ASSESSMENT:
*   ABCs: Ensure Airway, Breathing, and Circulation are stable.
*   Quick History and Physical Exam may focus on cardiovascular and neurological assessments.

2. RED FLAGS:
*   Try the CHESS mnemonic to identify patients at high risk for serious outcomes.

3. DIAGNOSTIC TESTING:
*   ECG: To assess for arrhythmias, structural heart disease, or ischemia.
*   Blood Tests: Blood glucose, full blood count (FBC), electrolytes, and cardiac enzymes if indicated.
*   Additional Testing: Consider echocardiography, Holter monitoring, or neuroimaging based on clinical suspicion.

4. DIFFERENTIAL DIAGNOSIS:
*   Narrow down the differential diagnoses. Consider both common and serious causes of syncope.

5. MANAGEMENT:
*   Admit high-risk patients (may apply the CHESS criteria and clinical judgment) for further evaluation.
*   Outpatient Management: For low-risk patients with a clear and benign cause of syncope, consider outpatient follow-up with appropriate referrals.

Are you missing something?

Understanding and recognizing specific conditions associated with syncope is crucial in the emergency setting. Below are some of the key conditions that should be on your radar.

1. HYPERTROPHIC CARDIOMYOPATHY (HCM):

HCM is a genetic condition characterized by thickened myocardial walls, often leading to obstructed blood flow and increased risk of arrhythmias.

Symptoms:
- Syncope, chest pain, dyspnea, palpitations; Symptoms are usually exertional.

Diagnostic Clues:
- ECG: Shows left ventricular hypertrophy (LVH) and may reveal Q waves.
- Echocardiogram: Demonstrates hypertrophy of the left ventricle, often with an asymmetrical septal bulge.

Management:
- Beta-blockers, calcium channel blockers, and in some cases, surgical interventions like septal myectomy or alcohol septal ablation.

2. BRUGADA SYNDROME:
A genetic disorder causing abnormal sodium channels in the heart, leading to a high risk of ventricular arrhythmias and sudden cardiac death.

Symptoms:
Syncope or sudden cardiac arrest, often during rest or sleep.

Diagnostic Clues:
- ECG: Characteristic coved ST-segment elevation in leads V1-V3, known as the Brugada sign.

Management:
- Implantation of an ICD (Implantable Cardioverter-Defibrillator) is the primary treatment.

3. LONG QT SYNDROME:
A condition (either inherited or acquired) characterized by prolonged ventricular repolarization, increasing the risk of torsades de pointes and sudden cardiac death.

Symptoms:
- Syncope, palpitations, seizures, or sudden death.

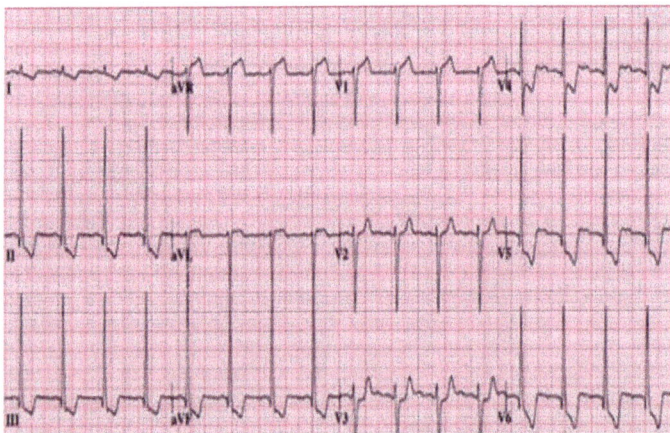

Figure 1.1 (left): Shown here is an example of an ECG with ST depression in the lateral leads, deeper S waves in the right precordial leads and tall R waves in the left precordial leads with T wave inversions indicating "strain pattern". These suggest left ventricular hypertrophy, a common feautre of **hypertrophic cardiomyopathy**

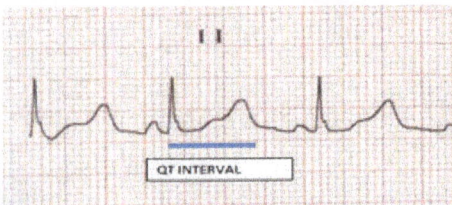

Figure 1.2 (lower left): Shown here is an example of **hypertrophic cardiomyopathy** with ST depression in the lateral leads, deeper S waves in the right precordial leads and tall R waves in the left precordial leads with T wave inversions indicating "strain pattern".

Diagnostic Clues:
- ECG: Prolonged QT interval, often >450ms.

Management:

- Beta-blockers, avoidance of QT-prolonging drugs, and ICD implantation for high-risk patients.

4. STATUS EPILEPTICUS:

A neurological emergency characterized by continuous seizures or >/=2 seizures without full recovery in between, lasting >30 minutes.

Etiology:

- Epilepsy, Learning difficulties, Encephalitis, Stroke, Brain tumor, Metabolic disturbances (i.e. hypoglycemia), Alcohol intoxication, Drug-related causes

Diagnostic Clues:

- Continuous/repeated seizures without regaining full consciousness.
- Bloods to assess metabolic (ie. blood sugar), electrolyte status;
- ECG; CT or MRI to identify structural brain abnormalities;
- Lumbar puncture (LP) if infection is suspected

Management:

- Treat hypoglycemia if present.
- IV Thiamine for patients with poor nutrition or alcohol abuse.
- Reinstate any withdrawn antiepileptic drugs (AEDs) and continue existing AEDs.
- Single dose of 4mg Lorazepam (or Diazepam 10mg IV)) as an initial treatment.

- If seizures persist after 10 minutes, give Phenytoin 18mg/kg (usual adult dose 1gm) diluted to 10 ng/ml in saline over 20 minutes or Fosphenytoin (15-18 PE equivalents).

5. COMPLEX PARTIAL SEIZURES (FOCAL SEIZURES WITH IMPAIRMENT OF CONSCIOUSNESS):

These are focal seizures that involve impaired consciousness. They often present with a combination of motor, sensory, autonomic, or psychic symptoms.

Symptoms:

Think of 5 As!

- **Aura**: Rising epigastric sensation, hallucinations
- **Absence**: Motionless state with a blank stare
- **Automatism**: Repetitive movements like lip-smacking or chewing
- **Autonomic**: Changes in skin color or other autonomic symptoms
- **Amnesia**: Memory loss of the seizure event

Diagnostic Clues:

- EEG: Shows characteristic spikes and wave patterns (BHZ Spike and wave).

6. NON-EPILEPTIC ATTACK DISORDER (NEAD):

NEAD resembles epileptic seizures but lacks the typical electrical disturbances in the brain. Up to 50% of cases of status epilepticus may actually be NEAD.

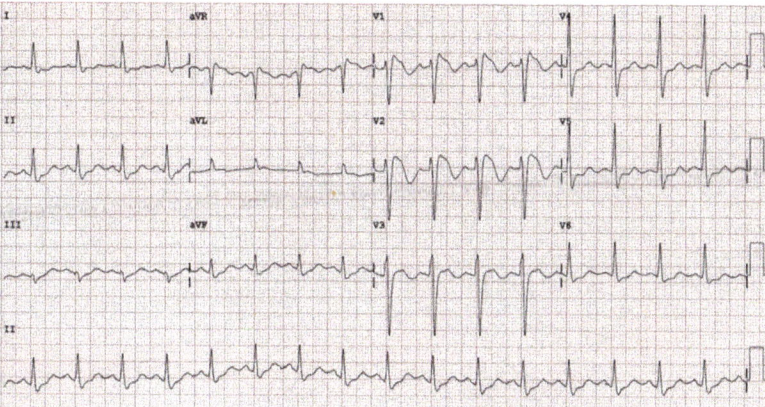

Figure 1.3
Coved ST segment elevation >2mm in >1 of V1-V3 followed by a negative T wave. This is called **Brugada sign.**

Diagnostic Clues:

- Careful clinical history and EEG monitoring can help differentiate NEAD from true epileptic seizures.

Useful mindmaps for brady-arrhythmias

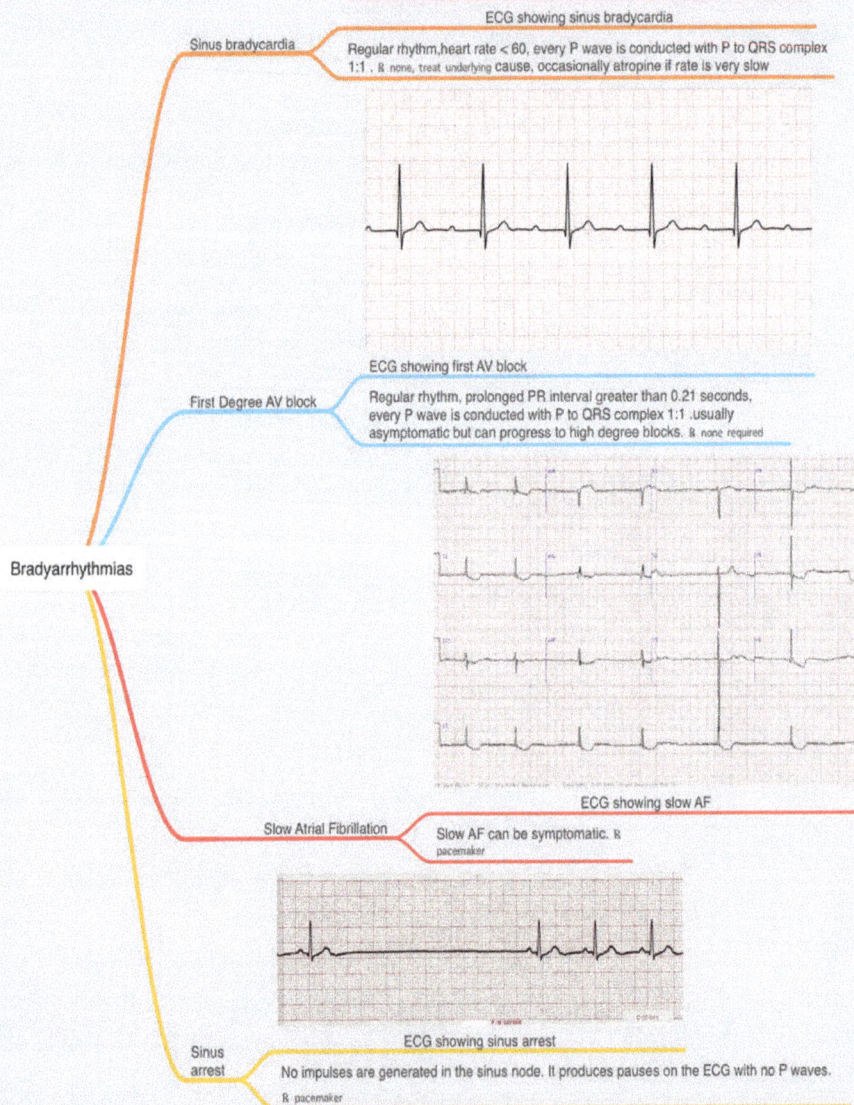

ECG showing sinus bradycardia

Sinus bradycardia

Regular rhythm, heart rate < 60, every P wave is conducted with P to QRS complex 1:1 . ℞ none, treat underlying cause, occasionally atropine if rate is very slow

ECG showing first AV block

First Degree AV block

Regular rhythm, prolonged PR interval greater than 0.21 seconds, every P wave is conducted with P to QRS complex 1:1 .usually asymptomatic but can progress to high degree blocks. ℞ none required

Bradyarrhythmias

ECG showing slow AF

Slow Atrial Fibrillation

Slow AF can be symptomatic. ℞ pacemaker

ECG showing sinus arrest

Sinus arrest

No impulses are generated in the sinus node. It produces pauses on the ECG with no P waves. ℞ pacemaker

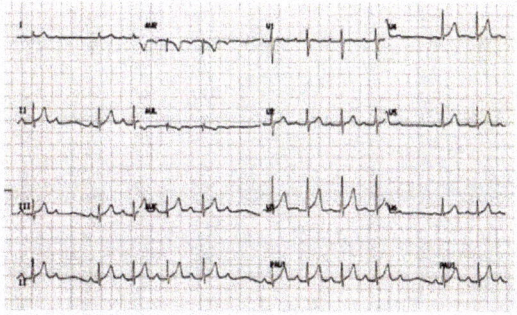

ECG showing Mobitz type 1 AV block

Mobitz type 1 AV block

. Irregular rhythm,
. delay in AV conduction with each successive impulse until an atrial impulse fails to be conducted due to impaired conduction in AV node .
. Usually benign and asymtomatic.
. R none required , rarely pacemaker

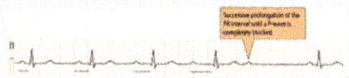

Succesive prolongation of the PR interval until a P-wave is completely blocked.

Dropped beat in Mobitz type 1
Also known as Wenkebach AV block

Mobitz type 2

. there is intermittent failure of conduction of atrial impulses without preceding progressive lengthing of the PR interval.
. The block is infranodal so the QRS complexes are usually broad. Commonly 2:1 AV conduction occurs.
. The atrial rate is regular with a constant P to P interval.
. This rhythm can be associated with Slow heart rate and sudden death.
. R: pacemaker, atropine

Brady arrthymias — **2 degree AV block**

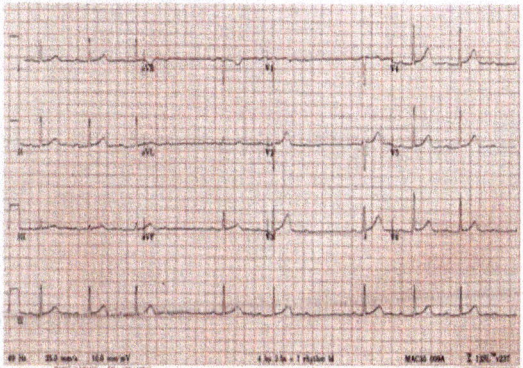

ECG showing type 2 Mobitz

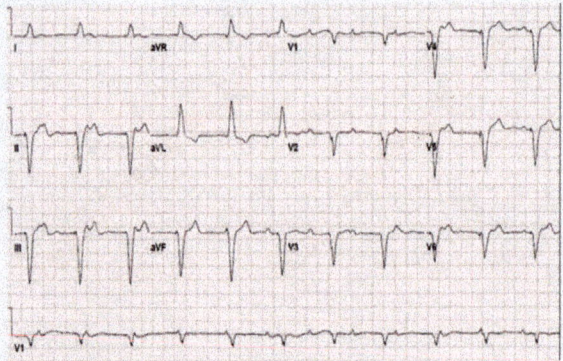

ECG showing complete heart block

Occurs due to complete blockade of impulses from atria to ventricles. The QRS complex can be wide or narrow depending on the block being infranodal or nodal. The rhythm is regular and p waves are regular. It can occur in association with Atrial fibrillation and atrial flutter.

к pacemaker

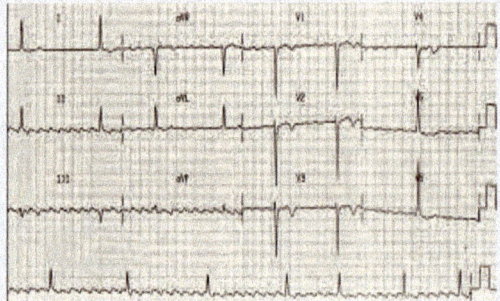

Atrial flutter with complete heart block

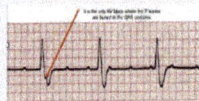

ECG showing buried P waves in the QRS complex

Brady arrthymias — Complete heart block

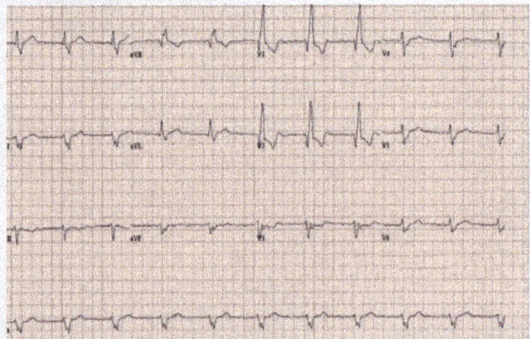

AF with CHB -AF becomes regular, no p waves visible

Differentiating causes of syncope

Features	Generalised fit	Vasovagal	Cardiac
Occurrence when sitting or lying	Common	Rare	Common
Prodromal symptoms	May occur	Typical	None
Tongue biting mm	Common	Rare	Rare
Urinary incontinence	Common	Uncommon	May occur
Injury	May occur	Uncommon	May occur
Facial colour	Flush	Pallor	Pallor
Post ictal confusion	Common	Uncommon	Uncommon
Focal neurological features	May occur	Never occur	Never occur
Return of consciousness	Slow	Faster	Rapid
Features	Automatism or hallucinations	Dizziness. Sweating, blurring of vision	Often none
Tonic -clinic movements	Prolonged twitching Occur within 30 seconds of onset	Brief twitching, can occur after 30 seconds of syncope	Brief twitching, Can occur after 30 seconds of syncope.
Duration	Longer duration	Short duration	Short duration
Confusion	Prolonged confusion and disorientation	Usually well orientated within 1-2 minutes	Usually well orientated within 1-2 minutes
Onset	Sudden, any position	Only occur sitting or standing , avoidable by change in posture	Sudden can occur in any position , not avoidable by change in posture
Immediate precipitating factors	Usually none	Emotional stress orthostatic hypotension, valsalva	Usually none
Frothing/hyperventilation	Common	Rare	Rare
Extremities	Extremities may be warm or flushed.	Usually pale and cold extremities	Usually pale and cold extremities
Post episode myalgia	Common	Rare	Rare

Blackout (TLoC) Causes

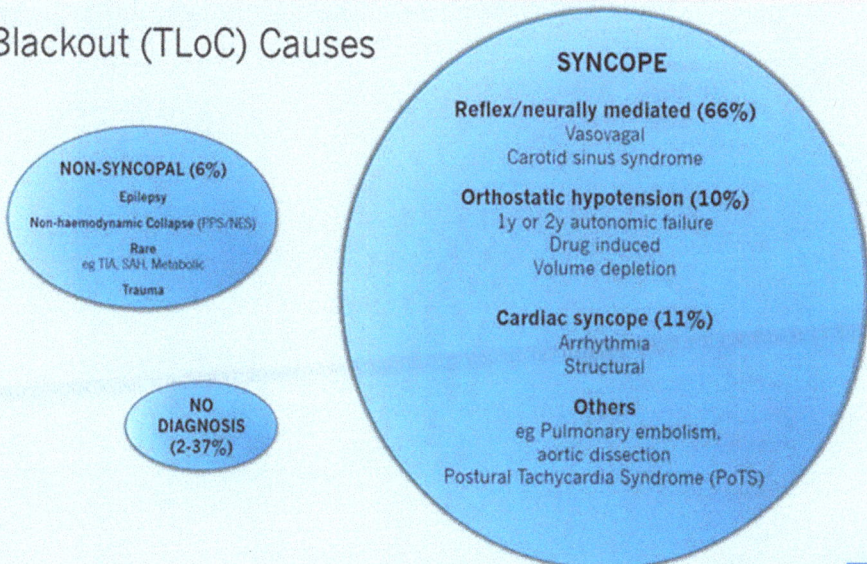

SYNCOPE

Reflex/neurally mediated (66%)
Vasovagal
Carotid sinus syndrome

Orthostatic hypotension (10%)
1y or 2y autonomic failure
Drug induced
Volume depletion

Cardiac syncope (11%)
Arrhythmia
Structural

Others
eg Pulmonary embolism,
aortic dissection
Postural Tachycardia Syndrome (PoTS)

NON-SYNCOPAL (6%)
Epilepsy
Non-haemodynamic Collapse (PPS/NES)
Rare
eg TIA, SAH, Metabolic
Trauma

NO DIAGNOSIS (2-37%)

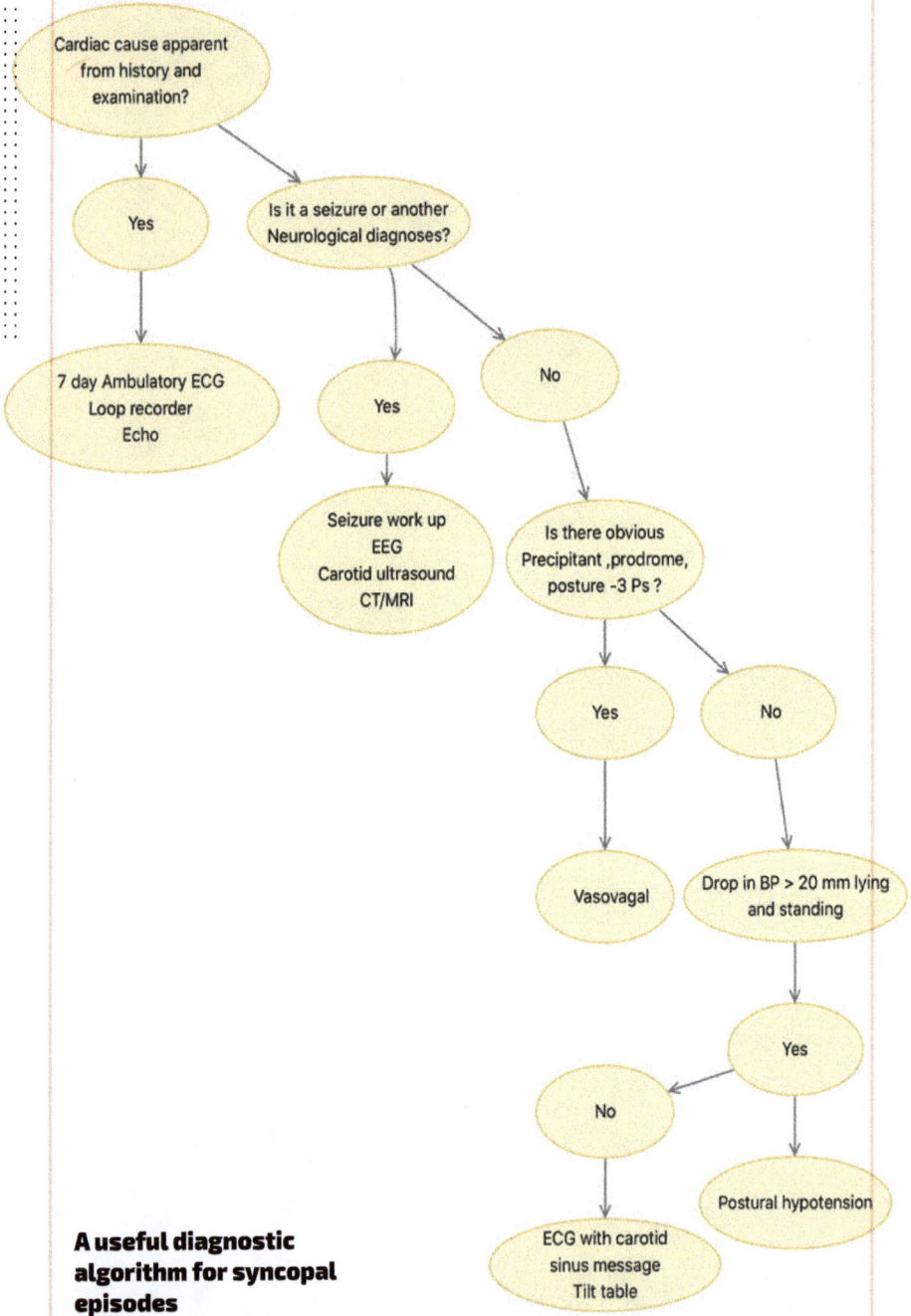

Cardiac cause apparent from history and examination?

Yes

Is it a seizure or another Neurological diagnoses?

7 day Ambulatory ECG
Loop recorder
Echo

Yes

No

Seizure work up
EEG
Carotid ultrasound
CT/MRI

Is there obvious Precipitant ,prodrome, posture -3 Ps ?

Yes

No

Vasovagal

Drop in BP > 20 mm lying and standing

Yes

No

Postural hypotension

ECG with carotid sinus message
Tilt table

A useful diagnostic algorithm for syncopal episodes

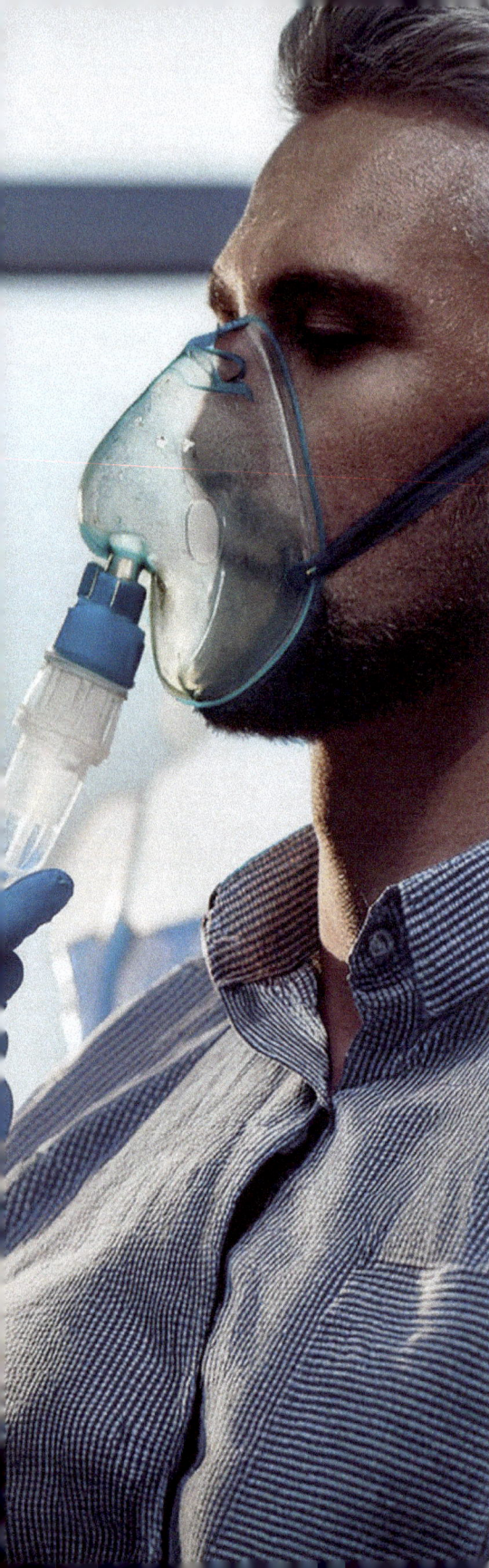

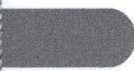

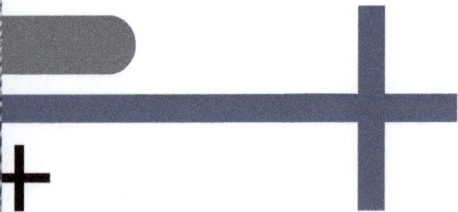

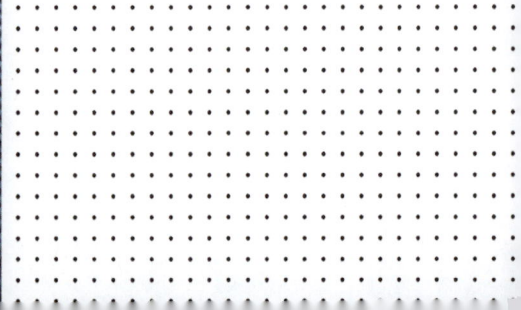

03

Shortness of Breath

Shortness of breath, or **dyspnoea**, is a common symptom with a wide range of underlying causes, from benign conditions to life-threatening emergencies. A systematic approach to history taking, physical examination, and targeted investigations is crucial to identify and manage serious diagnoses promptly. Recognizing red flags and clinical patterns can guide urgent interventions and improve patient outcomes.

Diagnostic sieves

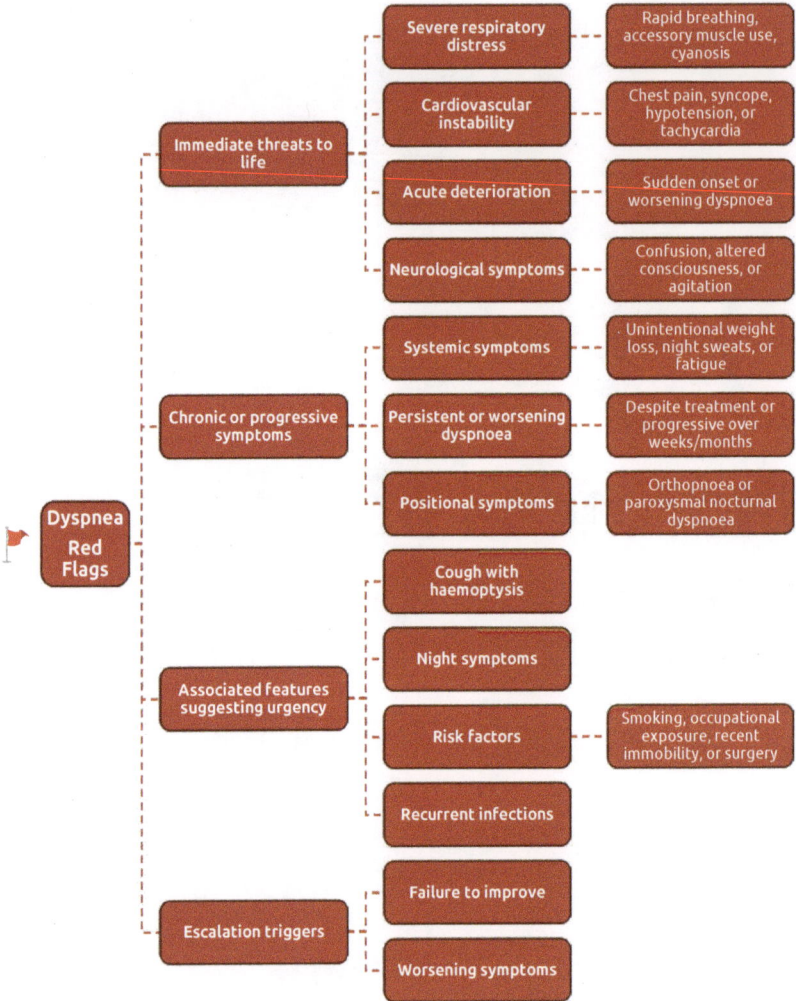

Dyspnea Red Flags

Immediate threats to life
- Severe respiratory distress — Rapid breathing, accessory muscle use, cyanosis
- Cardiovascular instability — Chest pain, syncope, hypotension, or tachycardia
- Acute deterioration — Sudden onset or worsening dyspnoea
- Neurological symptoms — Confusion, altered consciousness, or agitation

Chronic or progressive symptoms
- Systemic symptoms — Unintentional weight loss, night sweats, or fatigue
- Persistent or worsening dyspnoea — Despite treatment or progressive over weeks/months
- Positional symptoms — Orthopnoea or paroxysmal nocturnal dyspnoea

Associated features suggesting urgency
- Cough with haemoptysis
- Night symptoms
- Risk factors — Smoking, occupational exposure, recent immobility, or surgery
- Recurrent infections

Escalation triggers
- Failure to improve
- Worsening symptoms

History Taking - Important points

1. ONSET:
- Sudden: Suggests acute pathology, including pneumothorax, pulmonary embolism (PE), acute asthma exacerbation, acute heart failure, anaphylaxis, upper airway obstruction.
- Gradual: Suggests chronic or progressive disease, including COPD, interstitial lung disease (ILD), malignancy, anaemia.

2. PROGRESSION:
- Worsening over hours/days: Pneumonia, pulmonary oedema, uncontrolled asthma/COPD exacerbation.
- Worsening over weeks/months: Progressive ILD, malignancy, heart failure, pulmonary hypertension.

3. CHARACTER OF DYSPNOEA
- Exertional: Often seen in chronic conditions like cardiac failure or COPD.
- At rest: Indicates more severe disease, such as PE, severe heart failure, or pneumothorax.
- Positional: Orthopnoea in heart failure, paroxysmal nocturnal dyspnoea (PND) in cardiac failure, improvement when leaning forward in pericarditis or diaphragmatic paralysis.

4. ASSOCIATED SYMPTOMS
- Cardiovascular Symptoms: Chest pain (pleuritic in PE, pneumothorax, pericarditis; central and crushing in ACS or aortic dissection), palpitations in arrhythmias causing heart failure or ischaemia, syncope/presyncope in pulmonary hypertension, arrhythmia, or PE.
- Respiratory Symptoms: Cough (dry in ILD or early heart failure; productive in infection or COPD exacerbation), fever in infection or inflammatory conditions, haemoptysis (mild in PE, malignancy, bronchiectasis; massive in cavitating infections, vasculitis, malignancy), wheeze (expiratory in asthma/COPD; inspiratory stridor in upper airway obstruction).

- Systemic Symptoms: Weight loss in malignancy or chronic infections, fatigue/weakness in anaemia or chronic respiratory/cardiac disease, leg swelling in heart failure or DVT.

5. RISK FACTORS
- Pulmonary Embolism: Recent immobility (surgery, long-haul travel), hormonal factors (pregnancy, oral contraceptive pill, hormone replacement therapy), malignancy.
- Cardiac Disease: Hypertension, previous myocardial infarction, coronary artery disease, atrial fibrillation.
- Chronic Respiratory Disease: Smoking history (COPD, lung cancer), occupational exposure (asbestos, dust, chemical exposure).
- Infective or Inflammatory Conditions: Recent infection (pneumonia, tuberculosis), autoimmune conditions (rheumatoid arthritis, systemic sclerosis, lupus).
- Miscellaneous: Anaemia from dietary deficiency, chronic disease, or bleeding; neuromuscular causes like Guillain-Barré or myasthenia gravis.

6. PAST MEDICAL AND DRUG HISTORY
- Previous episodes of breathlessness or known conditions (e.g., asthma, COPD, heart failure).
- Medications that may exacerbate dyspnoea: beta-blockers worsening asthma or heart failure; amiodarone, methotrexate, or nitrofurantoin linked to pulmonary fibrosis.
- Recent hospitalisation could indicate surgery or immobilisation (risk of PE).

7. SOCIAL AND OCCUPATIONAL HISTORY
- Smoking history quantified in pack-years (relevant for COPD, lung cancer).
- Alcohol use and chronic alcohol-related conditions (anaemia, aspiration risk).
- Travel history for tuberculosis or PE risk.

Diagnostic sieves
■ □ □ +

Serious diagnoses to consider

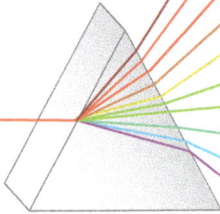

- Pulmonary Embolism (PE)
- Pneumothorax
- Acute Heart Failure/Pulmonary Oedema
- Asthma/COPD Exacerbation
- Pneumonia or Sepsis
- Upper Airway Obstruction
- Anaphylaxis
- Metabolic Acidosis (e.g., DKA)
- Interstitial Lung Disease
- Lung Cancer or Malignancy

! SERIOUS SYMPTOMS!

- **Pulmonary Embolism:** Sudden dyspnoea, pleuritic pain, haemoptysis, and leg swelling/DVT. Recent immobility/surgery.
- **Pneumothorax:** Acute, unilateral chest pain with dyspnoea. +/- reduced breath sounds on the affected side.
- **Acute Heart Failure:** Orthopnoea, paroxysmal nocturnal dyspnoea, frothy pink sputum, & bibasal crackles. History of hypertension/coronary artery disease.
- **Asthma Exacerbation:** Audible wheeze, chest tightness, and dyspnoea usually following identifiable triggers. "Silent chest" in severe cases.
- **COPD Exacerbation:** Dyspnoea, purulent sputum, and hypercapnic symptoms like confusion/drowsiness.
- **Pneumonia:** Fever, productive cough with purulent sputum, pleuritic chest pain. Localized crackles or consolidation.
- **Upper Airway Obstruction:** Stridor, difficulty swallowing, or choking sensation, commonly seen in anaphylaxis or foreign body obstruction.

! SERIOUS SIGNS!

- **Pulmonary Embolism:** Tachycardia, hypoxia, and a raised D-dimer. CTPA may show filling defects.
- **Pneumothorax:** Hyperresonance to percussion, absent breath sounds, and tracheal deviation in tension pneumothorax.
- **Heart Failure:** Elevated JVP, bilateral pitting oedema, and S3 heart sound.
- **Asthma/COPD:** Wheeze on auscultation, prolonged expiratory phase, or hyperinflation on X-ray.
- **Pneumonia:** Dullness to percussion, reduced air entry, and crackles or bronchial breath sounds.
- **Anaphylaxis:** Facial or laryngeal swelling, urticaria, and hypotension

- Occupational exposures to asbestos, silica, coal dust, or other chemicals.

Are you missing something?

- **Pulmonary Embolism (PE)**: Presents with sudden onset dyspnoea, pleuritic chest pain, tachycardia, and hypoxia. Haemoptysis or leg swelling may also occur. Prompt assessment using the Wells Score and D-dimer testing is essential. Confirm diagnosis with CT pulmonary angiography.
- **Pneumothorax:** Acute unilateral chest pain with dyspnoea and reduced breath sounds. Tension pneumothorax is a medical emergency requiring immediate needle decompression.
- **Acute Heart Failure (Pulmonary Oedema):** Presents with orthopnoea, paroxysmal nocturnal dyspnoea, and frothy pink sputum. Look for bibasal crackles and signs of fluid overload.
- **Anaphylaxis:** Rapid onset dyspnoea with stridor, urticaria, and hypotension. Requires urgent IM adrenaline and airway management.
- **Severe Asthma or COPD Exacerbation**: Dyspnoea with wheezing, accessory muscle use, and reduced air entry. "Silent chest" suggests impending respiratory failure.

Top tips

CLINICAL PATTERNS AND RED FLAGS
Red Flags for Cardiac or Respiratory Arrest:

- Profound hypoxia (SpO_2 <90% on high-flow oxygen).
- Inability to speak in full sentences.
- Cyanosis or altered mental status.

Approach and Risk Stratification

- **Pulmonary Embolism:** Use the Wells Score or PERC to estimate likelihood, followed by D-dimer or imaging.
- **Pneumonia:** Employ CURB-65 to assess severity and need for hospitalization.
- **Asthma/COPD**: Classify exacerbations as mild, moderate, or severe based on response to bronchodilators, oxygenation, and peak expiratory flow rate.
- Rapid bedside investigations include pulse oximetry, ABG, and portable chest X-ray.
- Use targeted blood tests (troponins, BNP, D-dimer) and imaging (CTPA, echocardiography) based on clinical suspicion.

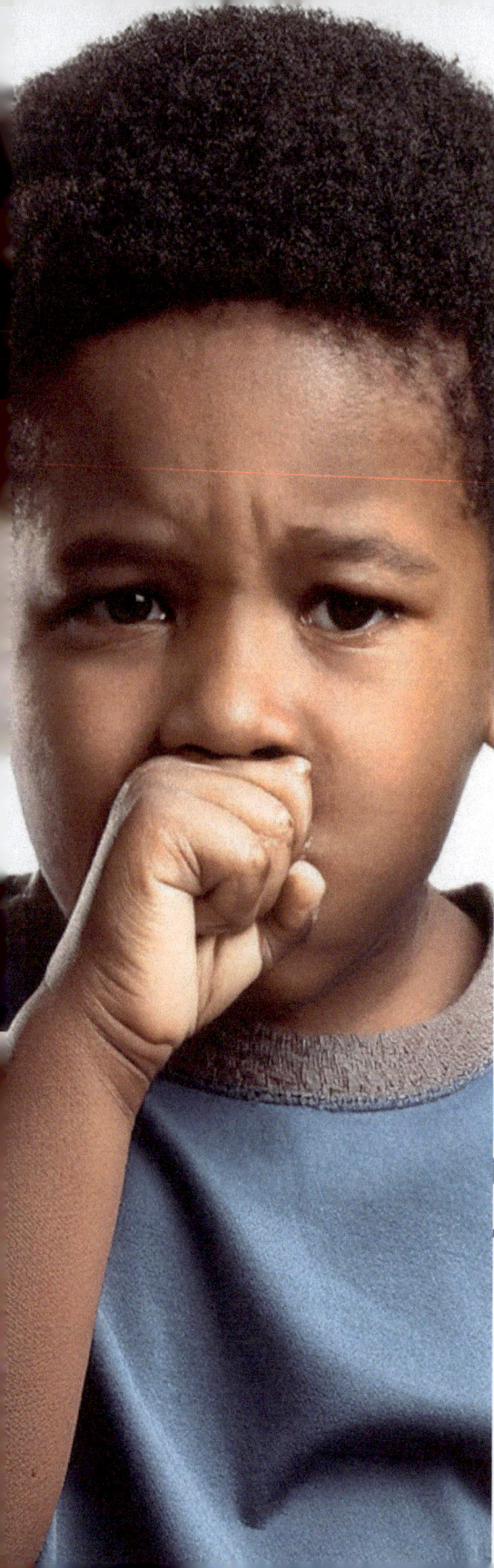

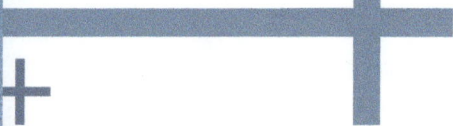

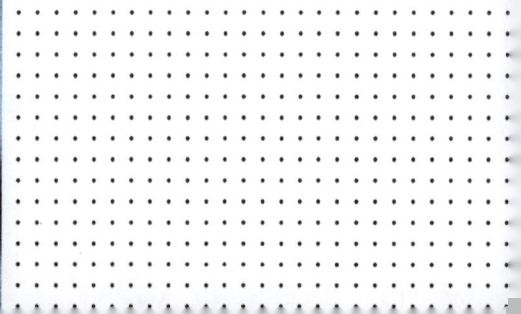

04
Cough

Cough is a reflex mechanism designed to clear the airways of irritants, mucus, and pathogens. While it is a common symptom, its causes range from benign, self-limiting conditions like viral infections to serious diseases such as lung cancer or pulmonary fibrosis. Effective management depends on identifying the underlying cause through a thorough assessment.

Diagnostic sieves

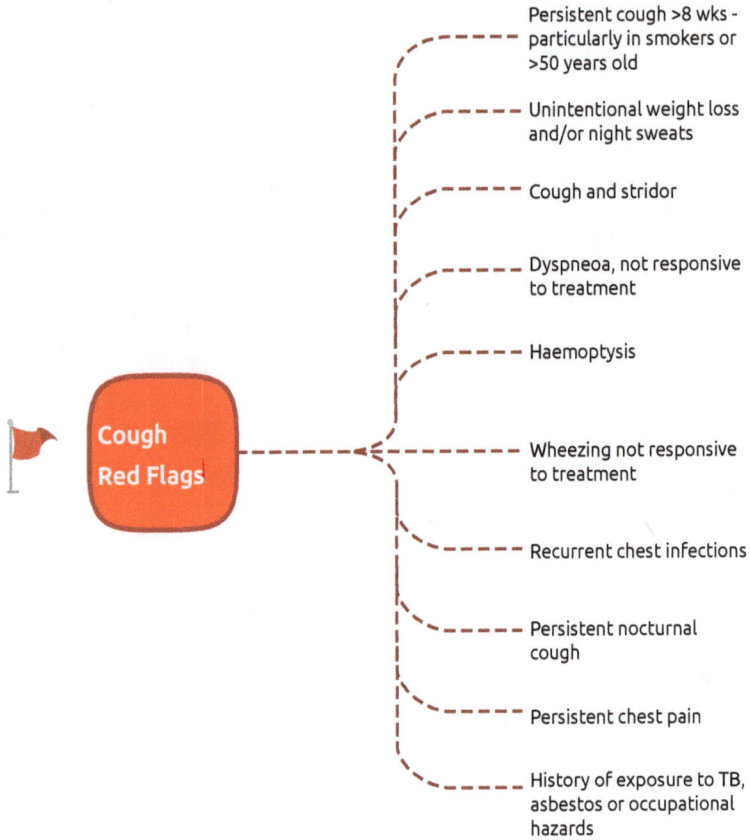

Cough Red Flags

- Persistent cough >8 wks - particularly in smokers or >50 years old
- Unintentional weight loss and/or night sweats
- Cough and stridor
- Dyspneoa, not responsive to treatment
- Haemoptysis
- Wheezing not responsive to treatment
- Recurrent chest infections
- Persistent nocturnal cough
- Persistent chest pain
- History of exposure to TB, asbestos or occupational hazards

Differential Diagnoses for cough

COMMON DIAGNOSES	SERIOUS DIAGNOSES
Respiratory tract infections	Lung Cancer
Asthma	TB
Rhinitis	Heart Failure
GORD	Laryngeal Carcinoma
COPD	
Bronchiectasis	

History taking

I. DURATION AND PATTERN

How long has it been going on?

- Acute onset (<3 weeks): Common causes include URTI, pneumonia, pulmonary embolism (PE), and pulmonary edema.
- Chronic cough (>2 months): Consider acid reflux (GERD), COPD, asthma, or pulmonary fibrosis.

Is it episodic or persistent?

- Episodic: More commonly seen in asthma, heart failure, and allergic rhinitis.
- Persistent: More commonly seen in COPD, pneumonia, and URTI.

2. CHARACTER OF THE COUGH

Is it worse at certain times of the day?

- Asthma: Worse at night.
- GERD: Worse at night or in the morning.
- Occupational asthma: Worse at work, better during holidays.
- Allergic rhinitis: Worse in the spring.

What is the nature of the cough?

- Chesty cough: Seen in pneumonia, pulmonary edema, and COPD.
- Dry or "trickle" cough: Common in asthma, ACE inhibitor use, and URTI.

Is it productive, and what is the color of sputum?

- Clear: COPD.
- Green: Suggests bacterial infection.
- Rusty brown: Indicative of pneumonia.
- Pink frothy sputum: Pulmonary edema.

3. EXACERBATING FACTORS

- Asthma: Triggered by exercise, emotion, laughing, or exposure to dust or cold weather.

- GERD: Coughing often occurs after eating.
- Pulmonary edema: Coughing may worsen when lying down.

4. ASSOCIATED SYMPTOMS

Ask about symptoms such as:

- Wheeze, hemoptysis, chest pain, breathlessness, fever, weight loss, night sweats, ankle swelling, or hoarseness of voice.

5. RISK FACTORS

- Smoking history: Assess smoking status and exposure to environmental irritants.
- Chronic respiratory conditions: Consider bronchiectasis, tuberculosis, or malignancy.
- Occupational or environmental exposure: History of exposure to TB, asbestos, or pets (e.g., birds at home).
- Postnasal drip history: Consider allergic rhinitis or sinusitis.
- Heartburn: Points to GERD.
- Flu-like symptoms: Suggests post-infectious cough.
- Use of ACE inhibitors: Consider drug-induced cough.

6. OTHER SPECIFIC FEATURES

- Cough associated with wheeze: Think asthma or congestive heart failure (CCF).
- Hoarseness: Suggests GERD, laryngitis, or postnasal drip.
- Frequent secretions in the throat: Consider postnasal drip or sinusitis.
- Chronic bad breath: Suggests chronic sinusitis.

Symptoms

Acute Cough (<3 weeks):

- Common causes: Viral upper respiratory infections (URTI), pneumonia, PE.

Subacute Cough (3–8 weeks):

- Common causes: Post-infectious cough, pertussis, asthma.

Chronic Cough (>8 weeks):

- Common causes: GERD, asthma, COPD,

Diagnostic sieves
■ ☐ ☐ +

Serious diagnoses to consider

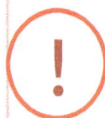

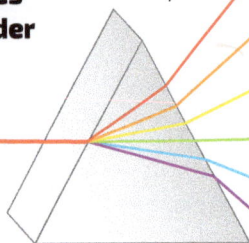

!

Lung or Laryngeal Cancer

Tuberculosis

Heart failure

Pulmonary Embolism

Interstitial Lung Disease

COPD

! SERIOUS SYMPTOMS!

- **Hemoptysis:** Suggests lung cancer, tuberculosis (TB), or pulmonary embolism (PE).
- **Severe or persistent chest pain:** May indicate pulmonary embolism, pneumonia, or pleuritis.
- **Unintentional weight loss or night sweats:** Red flags for malignancy or tuberculosis.
- **Severe breathlessness:** Suggests heart failure, interstitial lung disease (ILD), or pulmonary embolism.
- **Wheezing with cough:** Seen in asthma, COPD exacerbation, or foreign body obstruction.
- **Hoarseness lasting >3 weeks or dysphagia:** Indicates possible malignancy or laryngeal involvement.
- **Recurrent or chronic cough >8 weeks:** Suggests GERD, COPD, asthma, or bronchiectasis.

! SERIOUS SIGNS!

- **Cyanosis:** Indicates severe hypoxia, commonly seen in acute asthma, pneumonia, or pulmonary embolism.
- **Clubbing of fingers:** Suggests chronic lung conditions like interstitial lung disease, bronchiectasis, or lung cancer.
- **Tracheal deviation:** May indicate tension pneumothorax or significant mediastinal shift due to malignancy.
- **Stridor:** Points to upper airway obstruction from malignancy, foreign body, or laryngeal edema.
- **Dullness to percussion:** Suggests consolidation (pneumonia) or pleural effusion.
- **Use of accessory muscles or nasal flaring:** Indicates respiratory distress, as seen in asthma or COPD exacerbations.
- **Asymmetric chest expansion:** Suggests significant pleural effusion, pneumothorax, or lung collapse.

lung cancer.

Productive Cough:

- Green/yellow sputum: Likely bacterial infection.
- Rusty sputum: Pneumococcal pneumonia.

- Pink frothy sputum: Pulmonary edema.

Dry Cough:

- Common in asthma, GERD, ILD, and viral infections.

Serious Diagnoses to Consider

1. LUNG CANCER:
- Key Features: Persistent cough, hemoptysis, weight loss, hoarseness.
- Diagnostic Tools: Chest X-ray, CT scan, bronchoscopy.

2. TUBERCULOSIS (TB):
- Key Features: Chronic cough, night sweats, weight loss, hemoptysis.
- Diagnostic Tools: Chest X-ray, sputum culture, Mantoux or IGRA testing.

3. HEART FAILURE:
- Key Features: Orthopnea, paroxysmal nocturnal dyspnea, pink frothy sputum.
- Diagnostic Tools: Echocardiogram, BNP levels, chest X-ray.

4. PULMONARY EMBOLISM (PE):
- Key Features: Sudden onset dyspnea, pleuritic chest pain, hemoptysis.
- Diagnostic Tools: D-dimer, CT pulmonary angiography.

5. INTERSTITIAL LUNG DISEASE (ILD):
- Key Features: Dry cough, progressive dyspnea, fine crackles on auscultation.
- Diagnostic Tools: High-resolution CT scan, pulmonary function tests.

6. CHRONIC OBSTRUCTIVE PULMONARY DISEASE (COPD):
- Key Features: Chronic productive cough, dyspnea, wheezing in a smoker.
- Diagnostic Tools: Spirometry, chest X-ray.

Diagnostic Approach

Initial Assessment:
- History and physical examination with focus on red flags.
- Perform a chest X-ray for chronic or unexplained cough.

Specialist Investigations:
- Spirometry: For suspected asthma or COPD.

- High-resolution CT scan: For interstitial lung disease or suspected malignancy.
- Sputum analysis: For TB or bacterial infections.

Consider Bronchoscopy:
- Persistent hemoptysis, unexplained chronic cough, or suspected malignancy.

When to Admit

Massive Hemoptysis:
- ≥600 mL in 24 hours or ≥150 mL/hour.
- Associated respiratory distress or hemodynamic instability.

Severe Breathlessness or Hypoxia
Severe Chest Pain:
- Intense pain suggestive of acute causes

(e.g., PE, pneumonia).

Systemic Symptoms:
- Consider in fever.
- Sepsis, hypotension.

Top tips

- Always obtain a chest X-ray for smokers >40 years with persistent cough or hemoptysis.
- GERD is a common cause of chronic cough; consider empiric treatment in suspicious cases.
- Persistent nocturnal cough may indicate asthma or GERD.
- Look for occupational or environmental exposures in unexplained cases.
- Consider TB in at-risk patients

Are you missing something?

LARYNGEAL CARCINOMA

Don't miss the risk factors like smoking, alcoholism, male sex, age >60 years, lower socioeconomic status.

Common sites of origin are true vocal cords (glottis), and the supraglottic larynx while least common site is subglottic larynx.

Symptoms and signs are based on the involved position of the larynx- Hoarseness is common in early glottis cancers while airway obstruction is common in subglottic cancer. Supraglottic cancer often presents with dysphagia, airway obstruction and neck mass.

All patients who have hoarseness for 2-3 weeks should have their larynx examined by a head and neck specialist.

Laryngoscopy and endoscopy are the investigations of choice followed by CT.

Mneumonic for causes of cough

GASP AND COUGH

Gastroesophageal reflux disease

Asthma

Smoking/chronic bronchitis

Post-infection Sinusitis/post-nasal drip

Ace-inhibitor

Neoplasm/lower airway lesion

Diverticulum (esophageal)

Congestive heart failure

Outer ear

Upper airway obstruction

G I-airway fistula

Hypersensitivity/allergy

In smokers with new, persistent cough and red flags (e.g., hemoptysis or weight loss), prioritize early imaging to rule out malignancy.

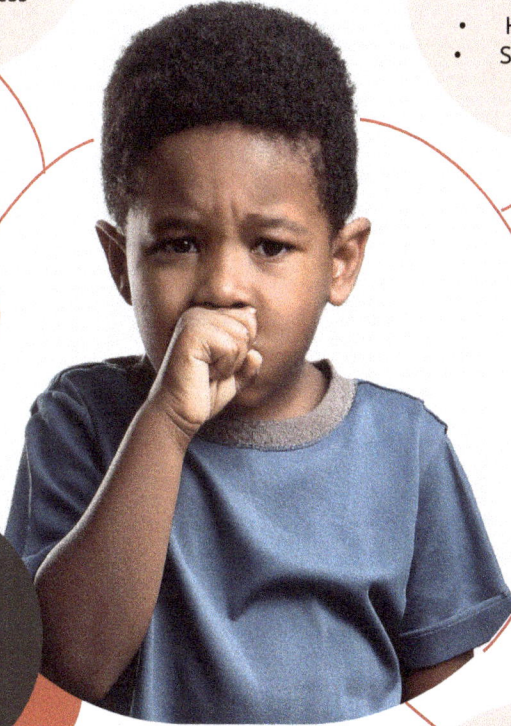

History
Symptoms suggestive of serious diagnoses:
- Haemoptysis
- Weight loss
- >8weeks duration
- Fever
- Breathlessness
- Chest pain

Exam
Signs suggestive of serious diagnoses:
- Clubbing
- Hypoxia
- Signs of sepsis

Serious differential diagnoses to consider

Differentials
Consider serious diagnoses:
- TB
- Malignancy
- Pneumonia
- Acute Asthma
- Pulmonary Oedema

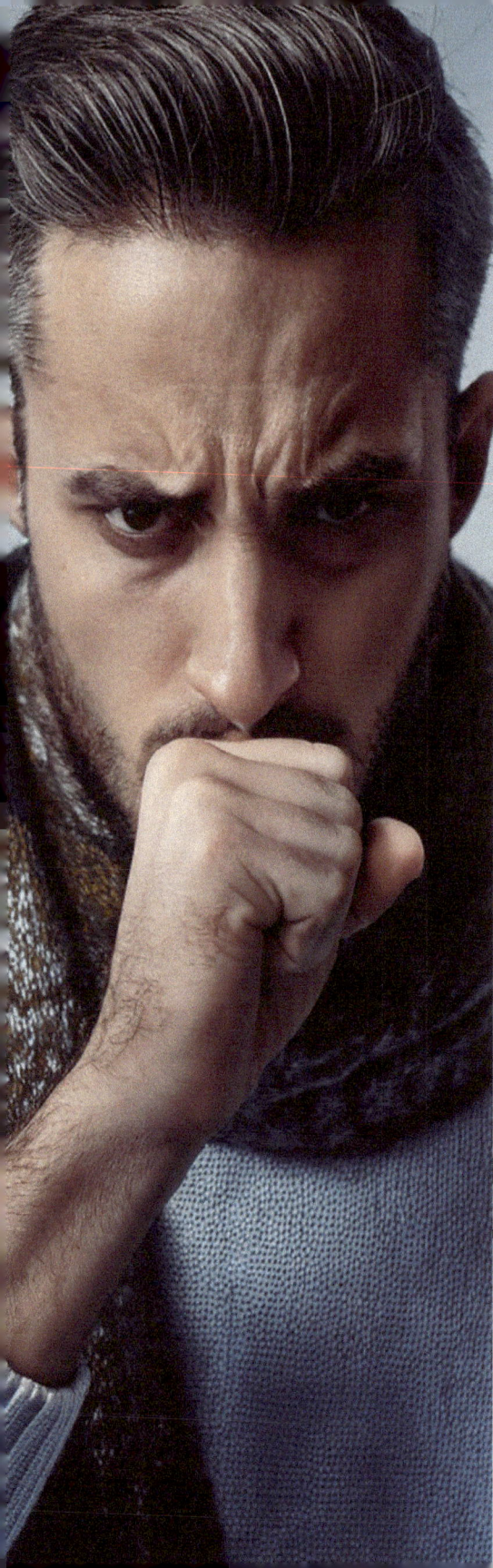

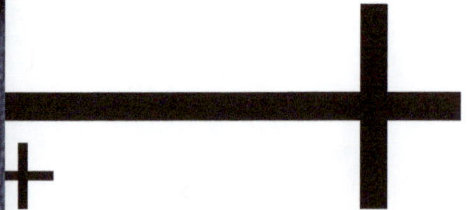

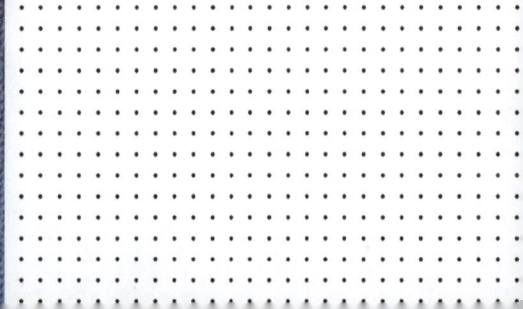

05
Haemoptysis

Haemoptysis refers to the expectoration of blood from the lower respiratory tract. It is a concerning symptom with causes ranging from benign infections to life-threatening conditions like malignancy or massive pulmonary embolism (PE). Accurate differentiation between true haemoptysis, pseudohaemoptysis (upper airway bleeding), and hematemesis (GI bleeding) is crucial. The volume of blood also determines urgency, with massive haemoptysis requiring immediate intervention.

Diagnostic sieves

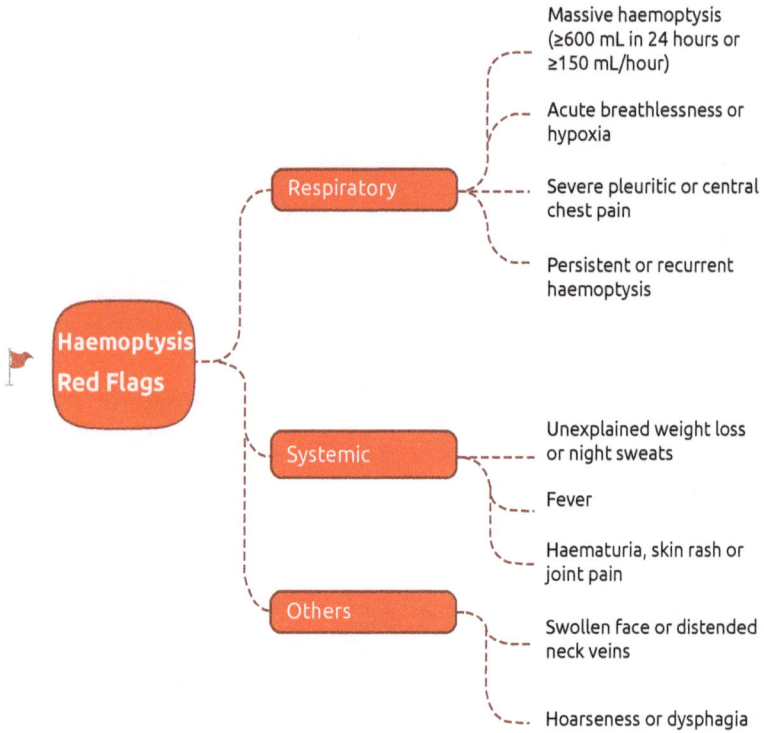

Haemoptysis Red Flags

Respiratory
- Massive haemoptysis (≥600 mL in 24 hours or ≥150 mL/hour)
- Acute breathlessness or hypoxia
- Severe pleuritic or central chest pain
- Persistent or recurrent haemoptysis

Systemic
- Unexplained weight loss or night sweats
- Fever
- Haematuria, skin rash or joint pain

Others
- Swollen face or distended neck veins
- Hoarseness or dysphagia

What really is acute PE?

Although PE is often described as having "sudden" onset, the PIOPED II study highlights a spectrum: 67% of patients report symptoms within seconds to minutes, while 87% experience them within hours. This variability challenges the oversimplified "classic" presentation and demands nuanced clinical judgment. Symptoms evolving over hours may still represent PE, despite appearing less acute. Clinicians must retain a high index of suspicion, use risk stratification tools, and carefully assess symptom timing to avoid missing this life-threatening condition. "Sudden" is a spectrum, not a fixed point.

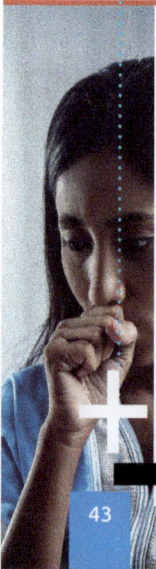

History taking: Key questions

1. ONSET AND VOLUME

How long has the haemoptysis been occurring?

- Short duration (days): Suggests PE, pneumonia, or severe infection.
- Chronic or intermittent (weeks to months): Suggests malignancy, bronchiectasis, or TB. Particularly in smokers, raises concern for malignancy.

How much blood is being coughed up?

- **Massive haemoptysis is concerning.** Life-threatening and often due to malignancy, TB, or vascular abnormalities.

2. RISK FACTORS

- Smoking, weight loss, chronic cough, or asbestos exposure (raises concern for malignancy).
- Recent chest infection.
- Immunocompromised state (e.g., ABPA, cancer).
- History of bronchiectasis, cystic fibrosis, or heart failure.

3. TIMING

- Haemoptysis after lying down: This may suggest upper airway origin.
- Coinciding with menstruation: Suggests endometriosis (ie. cyclical haemoptysis in thoracic endometriosis syndrome).

4. ASSOCIATED SYMPTOMS

- Acute breathlessness and chest pain: Suggests pneumonia or PE.
- Fever with weight loss: Suggests TB. Weight loss without fever: Suggests malignancy.
- Hematuria and epistaxis: Suggest vasculitis (e.g., Granulomatosis with Polyangiitis).
- Swollen face and distended neck veins: Suggests superior vena cava obstruction (associated with lung cancer).
- Persistent hoaresness: suggests malignancy.
- Sputum: Chronically producing large amounts of sputum suggests chronic bronchitis.

5. SYSTEMIC FEATURES

- Fever, arthralgia, skin rash, dyspnea: Suggest systemic lupus erythematosus (SLE).
- Sinusitis, hematuria, skin rash: Suggest Granulomatosis with Polyangiitis.

6. SPECIFIC HISTORY

- History of TB or HIV.
- Recent immobilization or surgery: Suggests PE.
- Use of anticoagulants: Suggests bleeding due to medication.
- History of bleeding tendency: Suggests chronic liver disease, coagulopathy, hrombocytopenia, or hemophilia.
- History of renal disease: Suggests Goodpasture syndrome.

Serious Diagnoses to Consider

1. LUNG CANCER:

- Key features: Persistent cough, haemoptysis, weight loss, hoarseness.
- Diagnostic tools: Chest X-ray, CT thorax, bronchoscopy.

2. TUBERCULOSIS (TB):

- Key features: Chronic cough, night sweats, weight loss, haemoptysis.

- Diagnostic tools: Sputum culture, Mantoux test, IGRA, chest X-ray.

3. PULMONARY EMBOLISM (PE):

- Key features: Acute dyspnea, pleuritic chest pain, haemoptysis.
- Diagnostic tools: D-dimer, CT pulmonary angiography.

Diagnostic sieves

■ □ ■ +

Serious diagnoses to consider

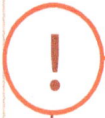

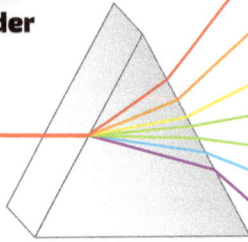

!

Lung Cancer

Tuberculosis

Pulmonary Embolism

Bronchiectasis

Vasculitis

Goodpasture Syndrome

Bacterial/Fungal Pneumonia

! SERIOUS SYMPTOMS!

- **Massive haemoptysis (≥600 mL in 24 hours or ≥150 mL/hour):** Life-threatening, often due to malignancy, TB, or vascular causes.
- **Acute breathlessness and chest pain:** Suggest PE, pneumonia, or pulmonary edema.
- **Unexplained weight loss or night sweats:** Raise concerns for malignancy or TB.
- **Hematuria and epistaxis:** Suggest systemic vasculitis.
- **Swollen face or distended neck veins:** Suggest superior vena cava obstruction, commonly seen with lung cancer.

! SERIOUS SIGNS!

- **Cyanosis:** Indicates severe hypoxia, seen in PE, massive haemoptysis, or pneumonia.
- **Clubbing of fingers:** Suggests chronic lung conditions such as bronchiectasis, interstitial lung disease, or lung cancer.
- **Tracheal deviation:** May indicate tension pneumothorax or significant mediastinal shift.
- **Wheeze or stridor:** Indicates upper airway obstruction from malignancy, foreign body, or edema.
- **Dullness to percussion and reduced breath sounds:** Suggest pleural effusion or consolidation.
- **Tachycardia and hypotension:** Signs of hemodynamic instability due to massive haemoptysis or PE.
- **Jaundice or pallor:** Suggests underlying liver disease or anemia contributing to coagulopathy.

4. BRONCHIECTASIS:

- Key features: Chronic productive cough with purulent sputum, recurrent infections. Diagnostic tools: High-resolution CT scan.

5. VASCULITIS:

e.g. Granulomatosis with Polyangitis

- Key features: Haemoptysis, nasal congestion, hematuria, skin rash.
- Diagnostic tools: ANCA testing, biopsy

6. GOODPASTURE SYNDROME:

- Haemoptysis, hematuria, renal impairment. Diagnostic tools: Anti-GBM antibodies, renal biopsy.

7. INFECTIONS:

e.g. Pneumonia, fungal infections (i.e. aspergillosis), severe infections

- Key features: Fever, productive cough, localized chest pain.
- Diagnostic tools: Sputum culture, chest X-ray.

Diagnostic Approach

Initial Assessment:

- History and Physical Examination: Assess hemodynamic stability and identify potential sources of bleeding.
- Basic Investigations: FBC, coagulation profile, renal function, and arterial blood gases (if hypoxia is suspected).

Imaging:

- Chest X-ray: First-line to identify infections, malignancy, or other abnormalities.

- CT Thorax: Gold standard for further evaluation.
- Bronchoscopy: For localization and biopsy in persistent or unexplained haemoptysis.

Special tests:

- Sputum Culture: For TB, fungal infections.
- Autoimmune Panel: ANCA, anti-GBM antibodies for vasculitis or Goodpasture syndrome

When to Admit

Massive Hemoptysis:

- ≥600 mL in 24 hours or ≥150 mL/hour.
- Associated respiratory distress or hemodynamic instability.

Severe Breathlessness or Hypoxia

Severe Chest Pain:

- Intense pain suggestive of acute causes (e.g., PE, pneumonia).

Systemic/decompensation features:

- Palor, tachycardia, fever, hypotension or sepsis

Are you missing something?

PULMONARY RENAL CONDITIONS.

The combination of new-onset respiratory signs, symptoms and abnormal investigations together with acute renal dysfunction could indicate a 'Pulmonary-renal syndrome'

While renal involvement may occur due to systemic illness such as severe sepsis, the term is reserved for new alveolar haemorrhage and Glomerulonephritis due to a Systemic vasculitis.

Classification

- Wegner's Granulomatosis : upper airway problems + positive c- ANCA/ PR3
- Microscopic polyngitis: C or P-ANCA positive
- Goodpasture disease
- Chaurg-strauss Syndrome

Differential Diagnoses using the Vitamin CDE framework

Category	Examples
V – Vascular	- Pulmonary embolism (PE)
	- Arteriovenous malformations (AVMs)
	- Aortic dissection (causing hemothorax and secondary haemoptysis)
I – Infectious	- Tuberculosis (TB)
	- Pneumonia (necrotizing or cavitary infections)
	- Fungal infections (e.g., aspergillosis)
	- Bronchiectasis-related infections
T – Toxicological	- Anticoagulants/antiplatelets (e.g., warfarin, DOACs, aspirin)
	- Inhaled toxins or irritants (e.g., caustic fumes, smoke inhalation)
A – Autoimmune	- Vasculitis (e.g., Granulomatosis with Polyangiitis, microscopic polyangiitis)
	- Goodpasture syndrome
	- Systemic lupus erythematosus (SLE) (rarely causing haemoptysis)
M – Metabolic	- Uremic pneumonitis (associated with chronic kidney disease)
	- Severe coagulopathies (e.g., liver failure, thrombocytopenia)
I – Idiopathic	- Idiopathic pulmonary hemosiderosis
	- Unexplained recurrent haemoptysis (after exclusion of other causes)
N – Neoplastic	- Lung cancer (most common serious neoplastic cause)
	- Metastatic disease involving the lungs
C – Congenital	- Cystic fibrosis (with associated bronchiectasis)
	- Hereditary hemorrhagic telangiectasia (HHT) (AVMs and recurrent bleeding)
D – Degenerative	- End-stage bronchiectasis
	- Chronic obstructive pulmonary disease (COPD)
E – Environmental	- Foreign body aspiration
	- High-altitude pulmonary edema (HAPE)

Clinical features

- Respiratory: haemoptysis, alveolar haemorrhage,Cough, breathlessness, Pleuritic chest Pain.
- Upper tract features: epistaxis , nasal congestion , sinusitis and septal perforation.
- Renal: hematuria, oliguria and renal failure.
- Systemic: malaise, lethargy, fever, weight loss, rash

Investigations

- Urine - positive dipstick test for blood and proteins
- FBC, UEC, CRP, ESR
- Autoantibodies : ANA, DNA, anti-GBM
- CXR - alveolar haemorrhage
- CT Sinuses
- Pulmonary function tests - increased KCO
- Tissue Biopsy

PULMONARY EMBOLISM

The annual incidence of Pulmonary embolism (PE) is 60-70/100,000 with half of cases occurring in hospital. In hospital mortality ranges from 6-15 %.

Clinical features

1. Breathlessness = 82 % of cases
2. Tachypnoeic = 60 % of cases
3. Chest pain = 49 % of cases
4. Cough
5. Tachycardia; Tachypnea and tachycardia are the most common signs associated with pulmonary embolism at over 50 % and 26 % respectively in all patients with PE.
6. Syncope = 10 % of cases; syncope has been found to be the *initial symptom* in only 5 % or fewer cases
7. Haemoptysis
8. Fever

Massive PE is highly likely if all the features are present

- *Collapse/hypotension*
- *Unexplained hypoxia*
- *Engorged neck veins*
- *Right ventricular gallop*

Investigations

- D-Dimer – if normal PE is excluded in low probability cases
- CTPA – 90 % sensitivity and 95 % specificity
- Echo
- V/Q scan

Remember that:

Elderly patients present less frequently with Dyspnoea or tachypnoea regardless of pre-existing cardiopulmonary disease.

Top tips

- Differentiate the Source: Ensure the bleeding is from the respiratory tract and not pseudohaemoptysis or hematemesis.
- Urgent Referral: Any case of massive haemoptysis or unexplained recurrent haemoptysis requires urgent respiratory or oncology input.
- Smokers with persistent haemoptysis will need an urgent CXR; consider lung cancer until proven otherwise.
- Consider TB in elderly, immigrants and those with risk factors
- No cause is found after extensive investigations in 20 % of cases

Mneumonic for causes of haemoptysis

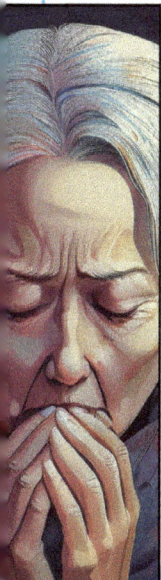

HEMOPTYSIS

Haemorhagic diathesis

Edema

Malignancy

Others (eg. vasculitis)

Pulmonary vascular abnormalities (PE)

Trauma

Your treatment

SLE

Infarction in lungs

Septic (infections)

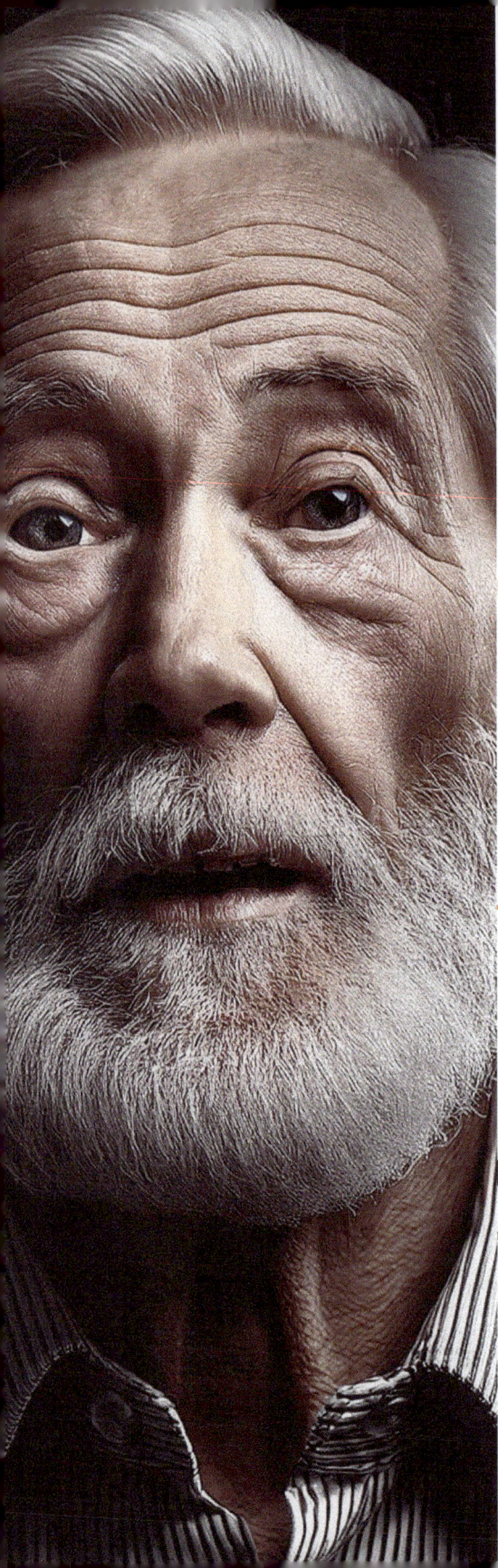

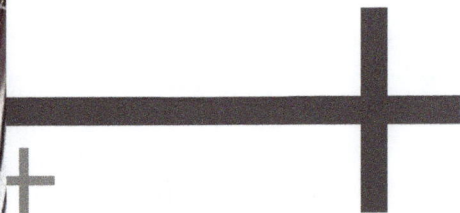

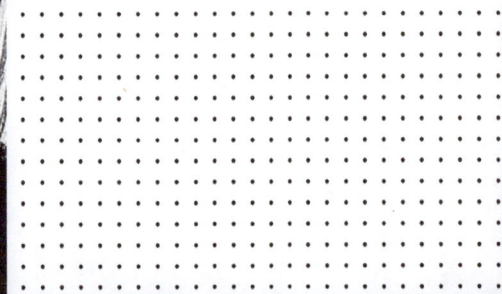

06
Hoarseness

Hoarseness, characterized by an abnormal change in voice quality, may arise from a wide range of causes affecting the larynx and vocal cords. While often linked to benign conditions such as acute laryngitis or vocal strain, persistent symptoms lasting more than three weeks should raise concerns about malignancy or structural abnormalities. A systematic evaluation, considering voice usage, systemic symptoms, and risk factors like smoking or gastroesophageal reflux, is essential for identifying serious underlying conditions and guiding appropriate management.

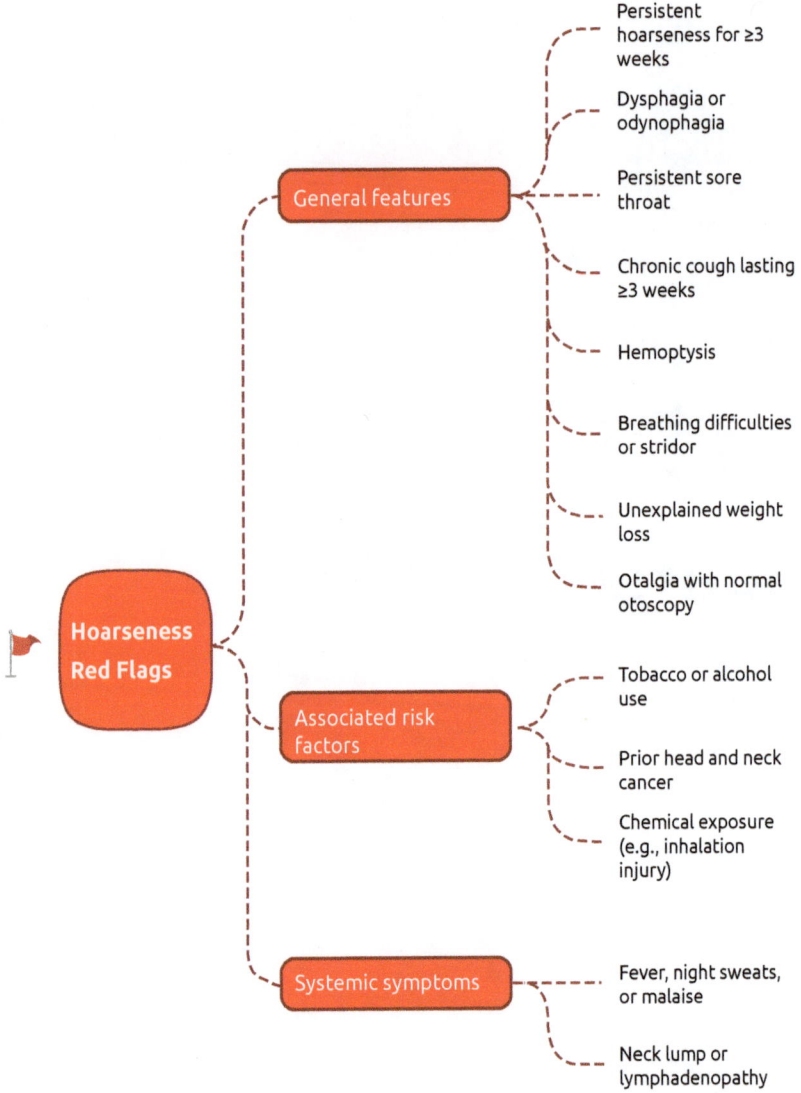

Hoarseness Red Flags

General features
- Persistent hoarseness for ≥3 weeks
- Dysphagia or odynophagia
- Persistent sore throat
- Chronic cough lasting ≥3 weeks
- Hemoptysis
- Breathing difficulties or stridor
- Unexplained weight loss
- Otalgia with normal otoscopy

Associated risk factors
- Tobacco or alcohol use
- Prior head and neck cancer
- Chemical exposure (e.g., inhalation injury)

Systemic symptoms
- Fever, night sweats, or malaise
- Neck lump or lymphadenopathy

History Taking - Important points

1. DURATION
- How long has the hoarseness been present? Persistent symptoms ≥3 weeks are concerning.

2. RISK FACTORS
- Does the patient have a history of smoking, alcohol use, or exposure to chemicals? These are significant risk factors for laryngeal carcinoma.

3. ASSSOCIATED SYMPTOMS
- Is there dysphagia, odynophagia, or aspiration? These may suggest malignancy or severe infection.

4. SYSTEMIC SYMPTOMS
- Are there fever, night sweats, or significant weight loss? Consider systemic diseases or malignancy.

5. NECK SYMPTOMS
- Is there a palpable lump or neck mass? Suggests possible malignancy or thyroid involvement.

6. VOICE USAGE
- Does the patient use their voice professionally or excessively? Vocal strain or functional causes may be relevant.

7. TRAUMA
- Any history of recent surgery, intubation, or vocal cord injury? Post-intubation hoarseness or trauma-induced damage should be considered.

8. MEDICATIONS
- Are they taking medications that can cause hoarseness (e.g., inhaled corticosteroids)?

9. RECURRENT INFECTIONS
- Any history of recurrent or chronic infections (e.g., sinusitis, laryngitis)?

10. GASTROESOPHAGEAL SYMPTOMS:
- Are there symptoms of GORD, such as heartburn or regurgitation? Chronic irritation from acid reflux may cause hoarseness.

Are you missing something?

- **Laryngeal carcinoma:** Persistent hoarseness for ≥3 weeks should be considered malignancy until proven otherwise.
- **Acute epiglottitis:** Rapidly progressing dysphagia or stridor warrants urgent evaluation.
- **Chemical inhalation injury:** Always ask about occupational exposures.

Top tips

CLINICAL PATTERNS TO NOTE
- Post-intubation hoarseness is often transient but may indicate trauma if persistent.
- GORD-associated hoarseness tends to be worse in the morning.
- Inflammatory conditions (e.g., laryngitis) are typically associated with recent infections or vocal strain

APPROACH TO DIAGNOSIS
- Always perform a thorough head and neck examination, including palpation for lymphadenopathy or neck masses.
- Visualize the larynx with nasendoscopy if symptoms persist beyond 3 weeks.
- Investigate with imaging (e.g., CT neck) for suspected malignancy or structural abnormalities.
- Consider thyroid function tests in patients with systemic symptoms suggestive of hypothyroidism

Diagnostic sieves

Serious diagnoses to consider

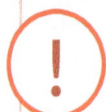

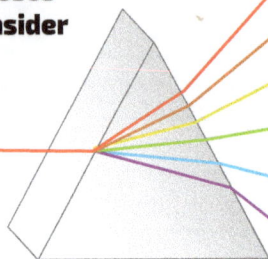

!

Laryngeal Carcinoma

Acute Epiglottitis

Chemical Inhalation Injury

Thyroid Malignancy with vocal cord involvement

Boerhaave's Syndrome (Ruptured Oesophagus)

Systemic diseases (e.g., Sarcoidosis, Granulomatosis with Polyangiitis)

! SERIOUS SYMPTOMS!

- Persistent hoarseness associated with:
  1. Dysphagia, odynophagia, or aspiration.
  2. Neck mass: Could suggest **laryngeal carcinoma or thyroid cancer**.
  3. Systemic symptoms (weight loss, fever): Consider **malignancy or systemic disease**.
- Rapidly worsening hoarseness with throat swelling: Suggests **acute epiglottitis or chemical inhalation**.

! SERIOUS SIGNS!

- Stridor or respiratory distress: May indicate **laryngeal obstruction or severe infection (e.g., epiglottitis)**.
- Neck mass or palpable lymphadenopathy: Concerning for **malignancy**.
- Visible lesion or abnormality on nasendoscopy.
- Unilateral vocal cord paralysis noted during laryngoscopy.

Differential diagnosis of hoarseness

Category	Examples
V – Vascular	Vocal cord hemorrhage, vascular malformation.
I – Infectious	Acute laryngitis, epiglottitis, pharyngitis, tuberculosis.
T – Traumatic	Intubation injury, vocal cord strain.
A – Autoimmune	Sarcoidosis, granulomatosis with polyangiitis.
M – Metabolic	Hypothyroidism (leading to vocal cord oedema).
I – Idiopathic/Functional	Muscle tension dysphonia, psychogenic causes.
N – Neoplastic	Laryngeal carcinoma, thyroid malignancy, metastases.
D – Degenerative	Age-related vocal cord changes (presbyphonia).
C – Congenital	Vocal cord paralysis (in children).

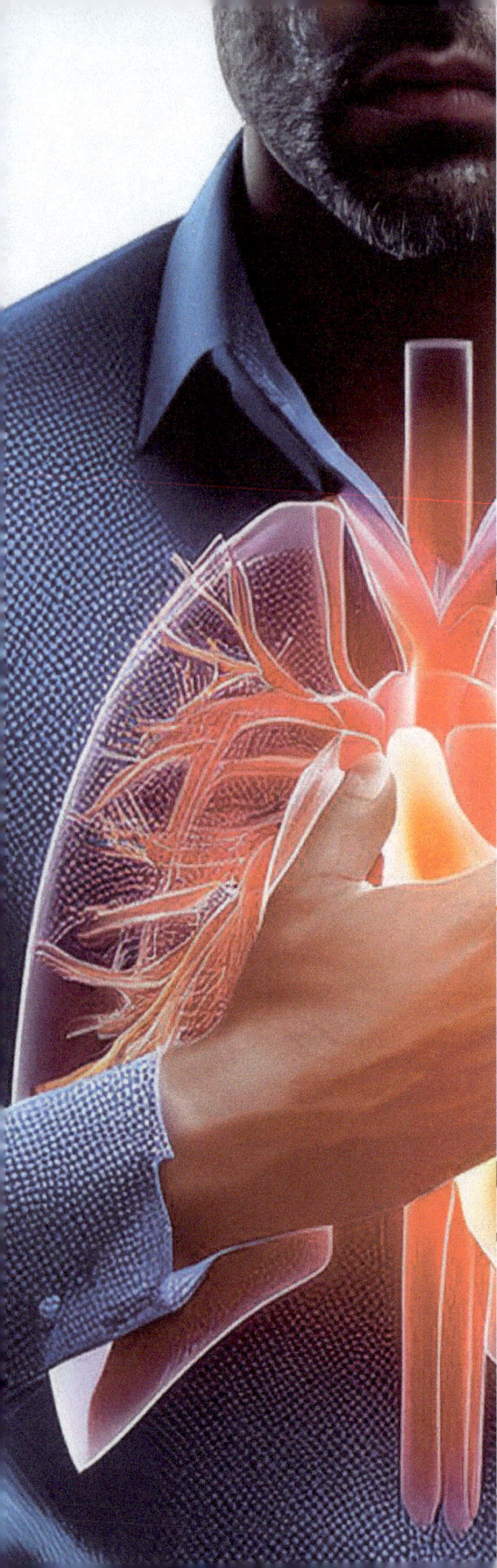

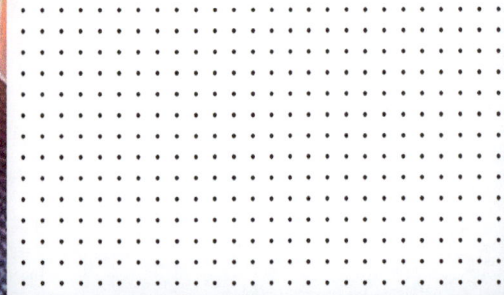

07

Dyspepsia

Dyspepsia refers to upper abdominal discomfort or pain that originates from the upper gastrointestinal tract. It encompasses a spectrum of symptoms, including bloating, early satiety, nausea, and epigastric pain. Common causes include gastroesophageal reflux disease (GERD), peptic ulcer disease (PUD), and functional dyspepsia, while serious conditions such as gastric or pancreatic cancer must be excluded. A systematic approach involving history, red flags, and targeted investigations ensures accurate diagnosis and management.

Diagnostic sieves

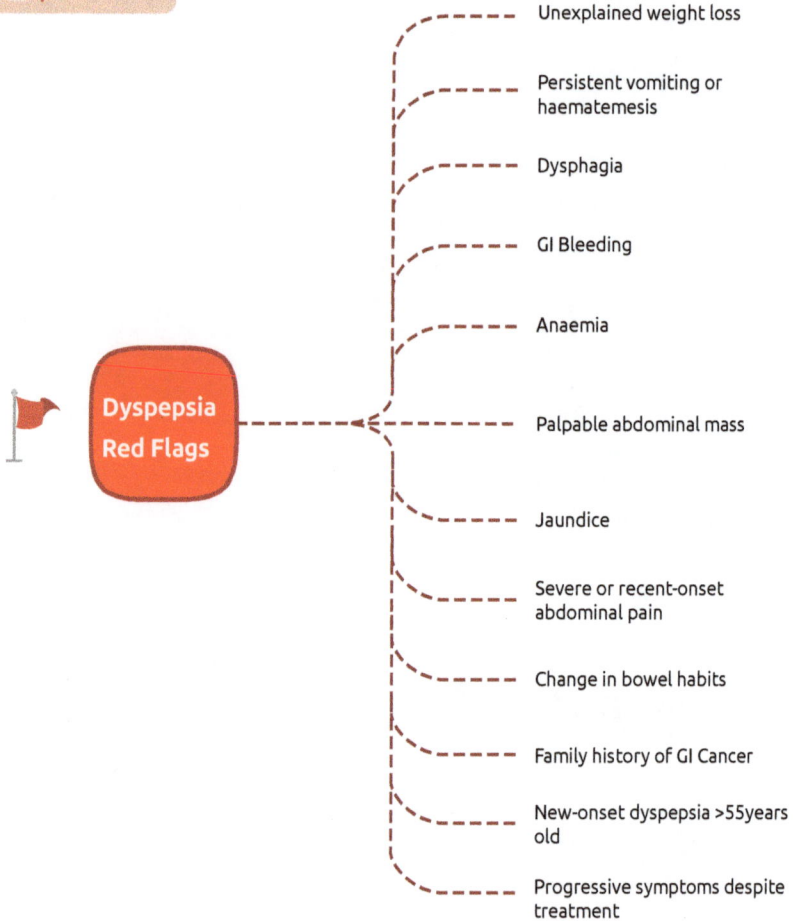

Dyspepsia Red Flags

- Unexplained weight loss
- Persistent vomiting or haematemesis
- Dysphagia
- GI Bleeding
- Anaemia
- Palpable abdominal mass
- Jaundice
- Severe or recent-onset abdominal pain
- Change in bowel habits
- Family history of GI Cancer
- New-onset dyspepsia >55years old
- Progressive symptoms despite treatment

Differential Diagnoses for dyspepsia

- Gastroesophageal Reflux Disease
- Peptic Ulcer Disease (PUD)
- Functional Dyspepsia
- Gastritis (H. pylori, NSAID-induced)
- Gallbladder Disease (Cholecystitis, Gallstones)
- Pancreatitis
- Oesophageal Cancer
- Gastric Cancer
- Functional Gastrointestinal Disorders (IBS, Postprandial Distress Syndrome)
- Lactose Intolerance
- Celiac Disease
- Infections (H. pylori, Gastroenteritis)
- Gastrointestinal Ischemia
- Drug-Induced Dyspepsia
- Gastroparesis
- Pancreatic insufficiency

History taking

1. CHARACTERIZING DYSPEPSIA

Onset:
- When did the dyspepsia begin?
- Helps determine if the symptoms are new or chronic.
- Has the frequency or severity of the symptoms changed over time? Changes may suggest a more serious underlying cause or progressive disease.

Nature of the Pain or Discomfort:
- Can you describe the pain or discomfort? (e.g., burning, gnawing, bloating, fullness, or cramping).
- *This can help differentiate between conditions like GERD, gastritis, and peptic ulcers.
- Is it localized to the upper abdomen or does it radiate elsewhere?
- Pain radiating to the chest, back, or shoulders may suggest cardiac causes or pancreatitis.

Timing of Symptoms:
- When does the discomfort occur? (e.g., after meals, in the morning, at night).
- Postprandial pain may suggest gastritis or peptic ulcers, while symptoms worse at night might indicate gastric ulcers or GERD.

Duration of Symptoms:
- How long do the symptoms last?
- Chronic symptoms lasting weeks to months could indicate a more serious condition, while acute, self-limited symptoms may be benign.

Triggers and Alleviating Factors:
- Do any foods or beverages make your symptoms worse? (e.g., fatty foods, caffeine, alcohol, spicy foods).
- *Certain foods can aggravate gastritis, GERD, or peptic ulcers.
- Do you notice any changes when you take antacids or over-the-counter medications?
- Improvement with antacids might suggest gastric acid-related causes (e.g., GERD, peptic ulcer).

2. RED FLAGS

Unexplained Weight Loss:
- Have you noticed any unintended weight loss recently?
- Unexplained weight loss can be a red flag for gastric cancer, pancreatic cancer, or malabsorption disorders.

Bleeding:
- Have you noticed any blood in your stool, black or tarry stools, or vomiting blood?
- Blood in the stool or vomiting blood may indicate peptic ulcer disease, gastric cancer, or variceal bleeding (especially in cirrhosis).

Dysphagia:
- Do you have difficulty swallowing food or liquids?
- Difficulty swallowing, or a sensation of food "getting stuck," may indicate oesophageal stricture or oesophageal cancer.

Jaundice:
- Have you noticed any yellowing of your skin or eyes?
- Jaundice can be indicative of pancreatic cancer, gallbladder disease, or liver pathology (e.g., cirrhosis).

Severe or Progressive Pain:
- Is the pain severe, or has it progressively worsened over time?
- Progressively severe pain could indicate a serious condition like gastric outlet obstruction or pancreatitis.

3. MEDICAL HISTORY

Previous GI Disorders:
- Have you had a history of ulcers, acid reflux, or other gastrointestinal conditions?
- A history of GERD, peptic ulcer disease, or gastritis increases the likelihood of these conditions recurring.

Recent Surgery or Procedures:
- Have you had any recent abdominal

Diagnostic sieves

Serious diagnoses to consider

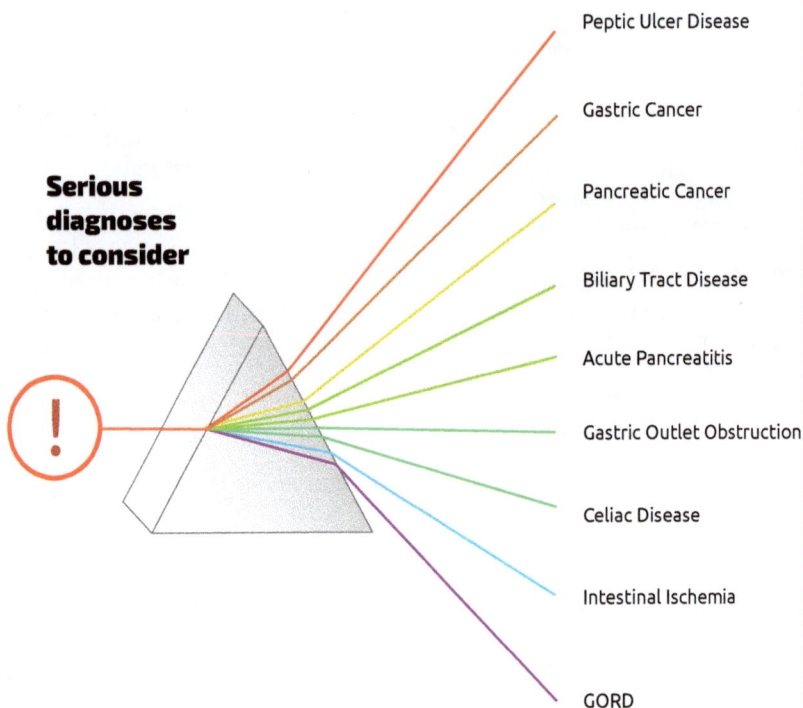

Peptic Ulcer Disease

Gastric Cancer

Pancreatic Cancer

Biliary Tract Disease

Acute Pancreatitis

Gastric Outlet Obstruction

Celiac Disease

Intestinal Ischemia

GORD

Causes of dyspepsia

Common	Uncommon
Alcohol gastritis	Abdominal wall pain (including incisional hernia)
Biliary disease	Food allergy
Food sensitivity	Gastric tumors
Functional	Referred pain (musculoskeletal, diaphragmatic, thoracic)
Gastroparesis	Vascular causes (mesenteric ischemia, median arcuate ligament syndrome, mesenteric venous thrombosis, aneurysms)
Helicobacter pylori gastritis	
Hepatitis	
Large hiatal hernia	
Medications[a]	
Pancreatic disorders	
Peptic ulcer disease	

[a] Nonsteroidal anti-inflammatory drugs, bisphosphonates, iron, corticosteroids, metformin, narcotics, antibiotics, and anticholinergics.

Culled from **Dyspepsia: A stepwise approach to evaluation and management By Deepika L. Chona**, MD et al; J Fam Pract. 2021 September;70(7):320-325 | 10.12788/jfp.0266

surgeries or procedures, such as gallbladder removal?

- Previous surgeries may contribute to gallbladder disease, gastric outlet obstruction, or post-surgical dyspepsia (e.g., after cholecystectomy).

Medications:

- Are you currently taking any medications, including over-the-counter drugs or supplements?
- Certain medications, such as NSAIDs, aspirin, or steroids, can increase the risk of peptic ulcers. Medications like antibiotics or PPIs may alter the gut microbiome or affect acid production.

Comorbid Conditions:

- Do you have any chronic medical conditions like diabetes, liver disease, or heart disease?
- Conditions such as diabetes (gastroparesis) or cirrhosis (with varices) can cause dyspepsia-like symptoms.

4. LIFESTYLE FACTORS

Dietary Habits:

- Do you consume large amounts of caffeine, alcohol, or spicy/greasy foods?
- Dietary factors can aggravate gastritis, GERD, or peptic ulcers.

Smoking:

- Do you smoke, or have you ever smoked?
- Smoking is a risk factor for gastric cancer, peptic ulcer disease, and GERD.

Alcohol Use:

- Do you consume alcohol? How much, and how often?
- Excessive alcohol use can contribute to gastritis, pancreatitis, and liver disease.

Stress Levels:

- Have you been experiencing a lot of stress or anxiety recently?
- Stress can exacerbate symptoms of GERD and gastritis.

5. FAMILY HISTORY

Gastrointestinal Conditions:

- Does anyone in your family have a history of gastric cancer, oesophageal cancer, or other GI conditions?
- Family history of GI cancers increases the risk of similar conditions in the patient.

Genetic Conditions:

- Are there any genetic conditions in your family, such as familial adenomatous polyposis (FAP), hereditary non-polyposis colorectal cancer (HNPCC), or Peutz-Jeghers syndrome?
- Family history of genetic conditions increases the likelihood of GI malignancies.

6. ASSOCIATED SYMPTOMS

Bloating, Nausea, and Vomiting:

- Do you experience bloating, nausea, or vomiting along with the pain?
- These symptoms may suggest gastroparesis, gastric outlet obstruction, or gastrointestinal infection (e.g., H. pylori).

Heartburn or Regurgitation:

- Do you have symptoms of heartburn, acid regurgitation, or a sour taste in your mouth?
- These are hallmark symptoms of GERD and can help differentiate it from other causes of dyspepsia.

Changes in Bowel Movements:

- Have you noticed any changes in your stool (e.g., constipation, diarrhoea, or blood)?
- Changes in bowel movements could suggest malabsorption, colorectal cancer, or GI bleeding.

Fatigue or Malaise:

- Do you feel fatigued or unwell in general?
- Fatigue may be associated with anaemia (e.g., due to GI bleeding) or a more systemic issue such as cancer.

Symptoms

1. UNEXPLAINED WEIGHT LOSS

- What it may indicate: Gastrointestinal cancer, particularly oesophageal, gastric, or pancreatic cancer.
- Why it's concerning: Significant weight loss without trying may suggest malignancy or malabsorption due to gastrointestinal diseases.

2. PERSISTENT VOMITING

- What it may indicate: Gastric outlet obstruction, gastroparesis, or gastric cancer.
- Why it's concerning: Persistent vomiting, especially with blood (hematemesis), can indicate a peptic ulcer, gastric cancer, or a gastric outlet obstruction that requires prompt diagnosis and treatment.

3. DYSPHAGIA (DIFFICULTY SWALLOWING)

- What it may indicate: Oesophageal cancer, strictures, or achalasia.
- Why it's concerning: Difficulty swallowing or feeling of food "getting stuck" in the chest suggests a potential oesophageal disorder that could be malignant.

4. GI BLEEDING

- What it may indicate: Peptic ulcer disease, gastric cancer, or variceal bleeding.
- Why it's concerning: Symptoms like hematemesis (vomiting blood), melena (black, tarry stools), or rectal bleeding could point to significant upper gastrointestinal bleeding, often associated with ulcers, varices, or malignancy.

5. ANAEMIA

- What it may indicate: Gastrointestinal malignancy (e.g., gastric cancer, colorectal cancer), peptic ulcers, or iron-deficiency anaemia due to chronic blood loss.
- Why it's concerning: Anaemia, particularly iron-deficiency anaemia, in the context of dyspepsia should raise suspicion for GI malignancy or a bleeding ulcer.

6. PALPABLE ABDOMINAL MASS

- What it may indicate: Abdominal cancer (gastric, pancreatic), or lymphoma.
- Why it's concerning: A mass may be

Mneumonic for alarm symptoms

ALARMS

Anaemia (iron deficiency), Age >60 yrs

Loss of weight

Anorexia, persistent vomiting

Recent onset of progressive symptoms

Melema/bleed or haematemesis

Swallowing difficulty/pain

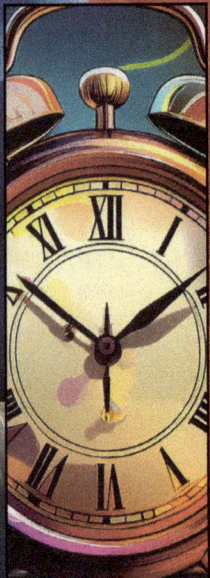

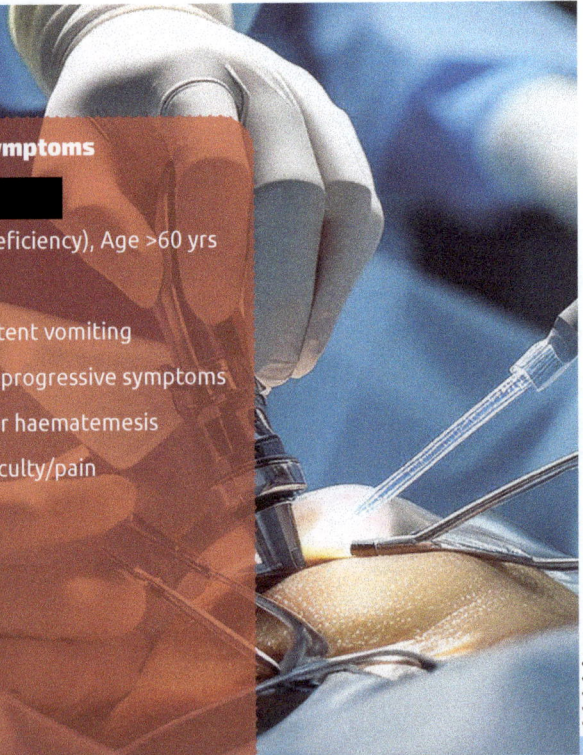

palpable on abdominal examination, which should prompt further investigation for malignancy or other serious conditions.

7. JAUNDICE (YELLOWING OF SKIN OR EYES)

- What it may indicate: Pancreatic cancer, gallbladder disease, or liver disease (e.g., cirrhosis, hepatitis).
- Why it's concerning: Jaundice with dyspepsia can indicate biliary obstruction or liver involvement, often linked to serious conditions like pancreatic cancer or biliary tract disease.

8. RECENT-ONSET OR SEVERE ABDOMI-NAL PAIN

- What it may indicate: Acute peptic ulcer disease, pancreatitis, or gastrointestinal perforation.
- Why it's concerning: Severe, sudden, or persistent abdominal pain can indicate a perforated ulcer, pancreatitis, or other acute GI conditions that require immediate intervention.

9. CHANGE IN BOWEL HABITS

- What it may indicate: Colorectal cancer or other serious GI conditions.
- Why it's concerning: A change in stool consistency, frequency, or the presence of blood in the stool (e.g., melena or haematochezia) may indicate a colorectal malignancy or a bleeding ulcer.

10. FAMILY HISTORY OF GI CANCER

- What it may indicate: A genetic predisposition to gastrointestinal malignancies (e.g., gastric cancer, oesophageal cancer, or colorectal cancer).
- Why it's concerning: A strong family history of GI cancers increases the risk of similar malignancies and warrants close monitoring.

11. ONSET OF DYSPEPSIA IN INDIVIDUALS AGED 55 OR OVER

- What it may indicate: An increased risk for gastric cancer or peptic ulcers in older individuals.
- Why it's concerning: In people aged 55 and older, new-onset dyspepsia (especially if it's a change from their usual pattern of symptoms) raises the suspicion for an underlying malignant cause such as gastric cancer or esophageal cancer.

12. SEVERE OR PROGRESSIVE SYMPTOMS

- What it may indicate: Malignant disease or serious peptic ulcer disease.
- Why it's concerning: If dyspepsia symptoms are progressively worsening or severe despite treatment, it could indicate a serious underlying pathology such as cancer, significant ulcers, or gastrointestinal obstruction..

Serious Diagnoses to Consider

- **Peptic Ulcer Disease (PUD)** - Can lead to bleeding, perforation, and gastric cancer.
- **Gastric Cancer** - Often diagnosed late, associated with weight loss, early satiety, and melena.
- **Oesophageal Cancer** - Progressive dysphagia, weight loss, and chest pain are key signs.
- **Pancreatic Cancer** - Weight loss, jaundice, and upper abdominal pain.
- **Biliary Tract Disease** - Gallstones, cholecystitis, and pancreatitis can present with dyspepsia.
- **Acute Pancreatitis** - Severe, acute upper abdominal pain and elevated pancreatic enzymes.
- **Gastric Outlet Obstruction** - Vomiting and fullness after eating, often due to ulceration or malignancy.
- **Celiac Disease** - Malabsorption, weight loss, and anaemia in patients with a gluten intolerance.
- **Intestinal Ischemia** - Severe abdominal pain, potentially leading to bowel infarction
- **Gastroesophageal Reflux Disease (GORD)** - Chronic reflux can lead to esophagitis

and Barrett's oesophagus, a precursor to oesophageal cancer.

Top tips

Example of Key Questions:

- How would you describe the pain or discomfort in your stomach?
- When did you first notice these symptoms?
- Do certain foods or drinks seem to make the symptoms worse?
- Have you lost weight unintentionally or noticed a change in appetite?
- Have you experienced nausea, vomiting, or difficulty swallowing?
- Do you have a history of ulcers, acid reflux, or other GI conditions?
- Do you have any family history of GI cancers or other GI diseases?
- Are you currently taking any medications, including over-the-counter treatments or herbal supplements?
- Do you consume alcohol or smoke? How much and how often?
- Do you have any associated symptoms like heartburn, bloating, or changes in your bowel movements?

Mneumonic for causes of dyspepsia

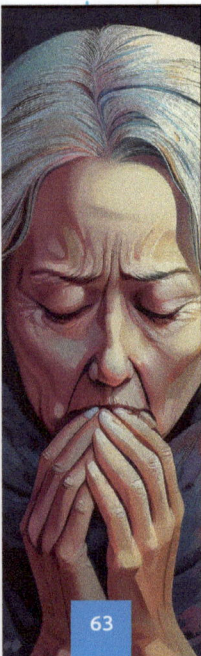

DYSPEPSIA

Vestibular/Vagal reflex (Pain)

Opiates

Migraine/Metabolic e.g. DKA

Infection

Toxicity (cytotoxic, digoxin)

Increased IOP/Ingested alcohol

Neurogenic

GI/Gestation

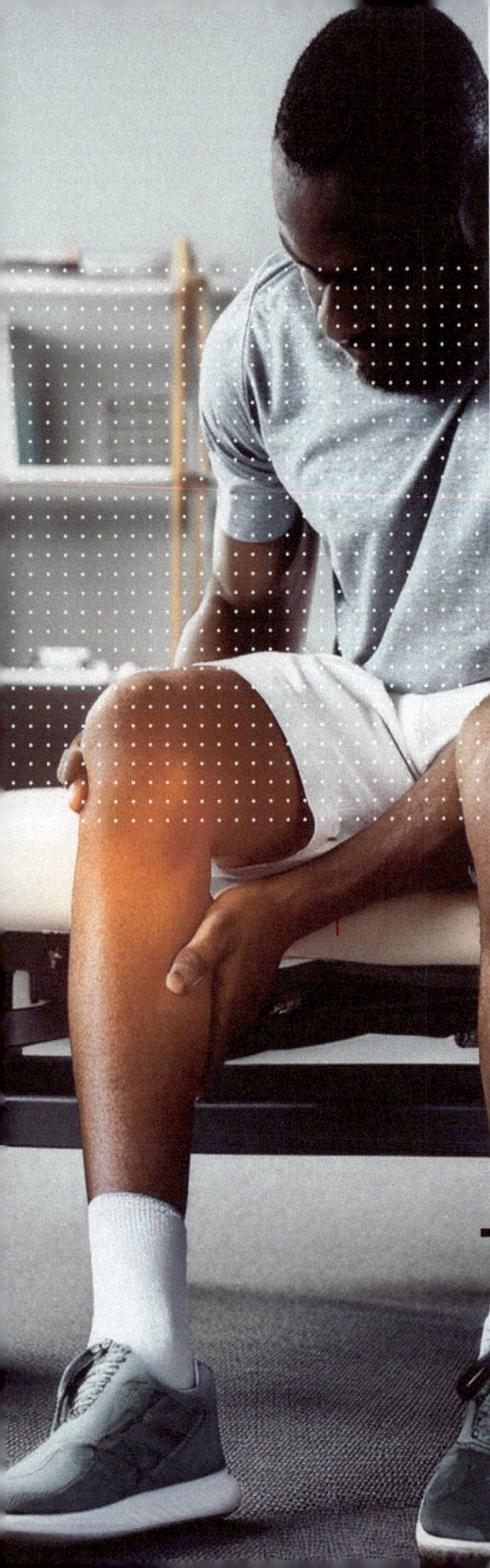

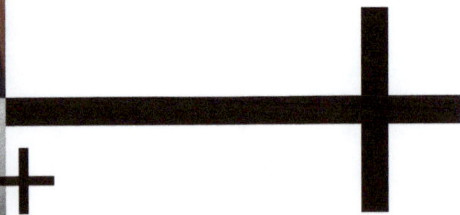

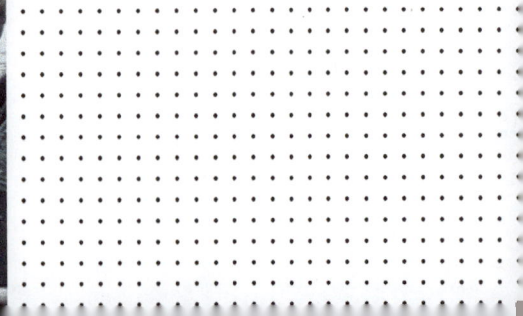

08

Swollen Calf

A **swollen calf** is a common clinical presentation with causes ranging from benign injuries to life-threatening conditions such as deep vein thrombosis (DVT) or compartment syndrome. It often results from localized processes like trauma, vascular obstruction, or infection but can also signal systemic illnesses. Early recognition of red flags and a systematic diagnostic approach are crucial for identifying serious causes and preventing complications such as pulmonary embolism or limb ischemia.

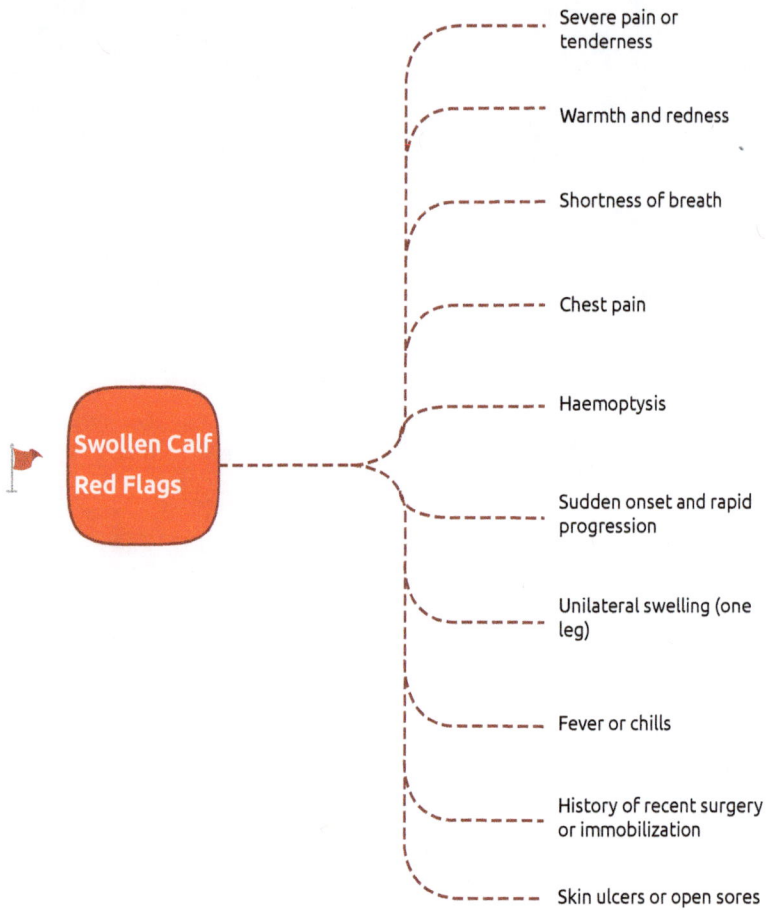

Swollen Calf Red Flags

- Severe pain or tenderness
- Warmth and redness
- Shortness of breath
- Chest pain
- Haemoptysis
- Sudden onset and rapid progression
- Unilateral swelling (one leg)
- Fever or chills
- History of recent surgery or immobilization
- Skin ulcers or open sores

History Taking

1. ONSET OF SWELLING:

When did you first notice the swelling in your calf?

- Helps determine the acute vs. chronic nature of the swelling.

Has the swelling come on suddenly or gradually over time?

- Sudden swelling might suggest trauma, DVT, or infection, while gradual swelling could indicate venous insufficiency, lymphedema, or chronic conditions.

2. TRAUMA OR INJURY HISTORY:

Have you had any recent trauma to the leg (e.g., fall, injury, or muscle strain)?

- Trauma could suggest a muscle tear, contusion, or fracture.

Did you experience any sharp, sudden pain in the calf after an injury?

- A sharp, sudden pain may indicate an Achilles tendon rupture or muscle tear.

3. PAIN:

Is the swelling associated with any pain?

- If so, where is the pain located and how severe is it? Pain can be a clue for conditions like DVT (pain in calf with swelling) or muscle strain (localized pain with swelling).

Does the pain worsen when you walk, stand, or move your leg?

- Pain exacerbated by movement might point toward a muscle injury, DVT, or tendinopathy.

Is the pain described as dull, throbbing, or sharp?

- Sharp pain could indicate a rupture or tear (e.g., Achilles tendon), whereas a dull ache might suggest venous insufficiency or mild muscle strain.

4. SKIN CHANGES:

Has the skin over the swollen area turned red, warm, or shiny?

- These signs may indicate infection (e.g., cellulitis) or DVT.

Do you have any fever or chills associated with the swelling?

- Fever and chills could suggest an infectious cause like cellulitis or osteomyelitis.

Have you noticed any colour changes in the skin (e.g., brown or purple discoloration)?

- Skin discoloration could be related to venous insufficiency or chronic oedema.

5. SWELLING CHARACTERISTICS:

Is the swelling unilateral (one leg) or bilateral (both legs)?

- Unilateral swelling may suggest DVT, infection, or trauma, while bilateral swelling is more often seen in venous insufficiency, lymphedema, or heart/kidney failure.

Does the swelling improve with elevation or worsen throughout the day?

- Improvement with elevation suggests venous insufficiency or lymphedema, while worsening with the day may indicate DVT or other acute causes.

Is the swelling pitting (can you leave a depression when you press on the swollen area)?

- Pitting oedema is more common with venous insufficiency, heart failure, or lymphedema. Non-pitting oedema might suggest a more chronic or inflammatory condition.

6. MEDICAL AND SURGICAL HISTORY:

Do you have a history of blood clots, heart disease, or any clotting disorders (e.g., deep vein thrombosis)?

- A history of DVT or clotting disorders increases the likelihood of a recurrent clot or venous insufficiency.

Have you had recent surgery or immobilization (e.g., bed rest, prolonged sitting, or

Serious diagnoses to consider

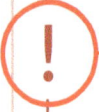

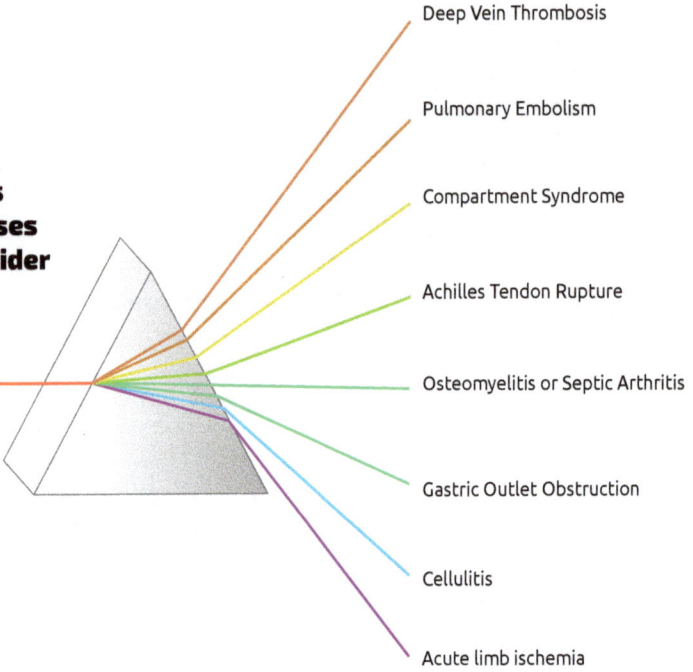

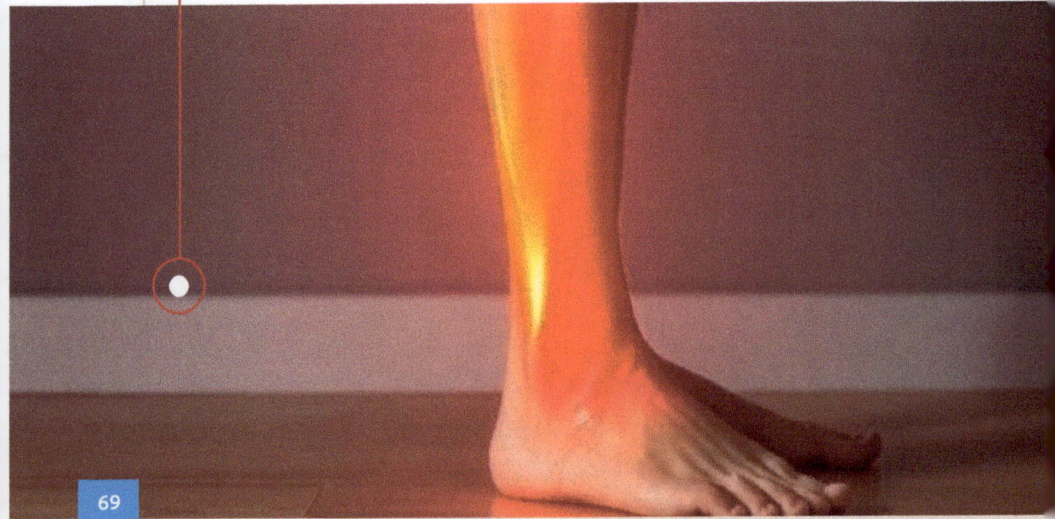

Deep Vein Thrombosis

Pulmonary Embolism

Compartment Syndrome

Achilles Tendon Rupture

Osteomyelitis or Septic Arthritis

Gastric Outlet Obstruction

Cellulitis

Acute limb ischemia

recent knee or hip surgery)?

- Recent immobility is a key risk factor for DVT and may lead to venous stasis and swelling.

Do you have a history of varicose veins, or any previous issues with swelling in your legs?

- Chronic venous insufficiency may present with recurrent swelling and skin changes.

Have you had any recent treatments or surgeries that could have impacted your lymphatic system (e.g., cancer treatments, lymph node removal)?

- Lymphedema, particularly following cancer surgery (e.g., mastectomy), could cause swelling in one or both legs.

7. RISK FACTORS FOR DVT OR PE:

Have you recently been on a long flight or car trip (long periods of sitting)?

- Prolonged immobility is a known risk factor for DVT.

Are you taking any medications that increase your risk for clotting (e.g., birth control pills, hormone replacement therapy, or anticoagulants)?

- Oral contraceptives, hormone therapy, or certain medications can increase the risk of DVT or clot formation.

Do you have a history of cancer, obesity, or other conditions that increase the risk for DVT?

- Cancer, especially with metastatic disease, and obesity are significant risk factors for thrombosis.

8. ASSOCIATED SYSTEMIC SYMPTOMS:

Have you noticed any recent shortness of breath, chest pain, or coughing, especially if the swelling is only in one leg?

- These symptoms could point toward a pulmonary embolism (PE) if a clot from the calf travels to the lungs.

Do you have a history of heart failure, kidney disease, or liver disease?

- Systemic conditions like heart failure, renal disease, or cirrhosis can cause bilateral leg swelling due to fluid retention (oedema).

9. ASSOCIATED MEDICAL CONDITIONS:

Do you have a history of diabetes, hypertension, or other chronic conditions that might affect circulation?

- Conditions like diabetes and hypertension can affect vascular health and predispose to complications like DVT, venous insufficiency, or peripheral artery disease (PAD).

Are you experiencing any generalized fatigue, malaise, or unexplained weight loss?

- These symptoms might be seen in systemic infections, cancer, or chronic inflammatory diseases.

10. LIFESTYLE AND ACTIVITY:

What is your typical level of activity? Have you had any changes in your exercise or physical activity recently?

- Changes in activity or overexertion could contribute to muscle injury or exertional compartment syndrome.

Do you stand or sit for long periods of time (e.g., job-related factors)?

- Prolonged sitting or standing (common in office workers or people who work on their feet all day) can predispose to venous insufficiency or DVT.

11. MEDICATIONS:

Are you currently taking any medications (including over-the-counter drugs, supplements, or herbal treatments)?

- Certain medications, such as corticosteroids, calcium channel blockers, or diuretics, can cause fluid retention or affect circulation and contribute to swelling.

Differential Diagnoses

I. DEEP VEIN THROMBOSIS (DVT)

A blood clot that forms in the deep veins of the leg, commonly in the calf.

- Key Features: Unilateral swelling, pain, warmth, redness, a feeling of heaviness, and sometimes tenderness. The swelling typically worsens over time.
- Risk Factors: Recent surgery, immobility, long travel, history of clotting disorders, use of oral contraceptives, or cancer.
- Diagnostic Tests: D-dimer test (initial screening), ultrasound (definitive diagnosis).

2. PULMONARY EMBOLISM (PE)

A blockage in one of the pulmonary arteries in the lungs, often caused by a clot originating from the lower extremities.

- Key Features: Sudden shortness of breath, chest pain (sharp, pleuritic), rapid heart rate, coughing (possibly with blood), light-headedness or fainting.
- Risk Factors: History of DVT, immobilization, surgery, or trauma.
- Diagnostic Tests: CT pulmonary angiography, ventilation/perfusion (V/Q) scan, D-dimer.

3. CELLULITIS

A bacterial infection of the skin and underlying soft tissues.

- Key Features: Swelling, redness, warmth, and tenderness over the affected area. The skin may appear shiny, and there may be fever and chills.
- Risk Factors: Diabetes, immunocompromised states, lymphedema, trauma to the skin.
- Diagnostic Tests: Clinical diagnosis (based on symptoms), occasionally culture or ultrasound to rule out abscess or deeper infections.

4. VENOUS INSUFFICIENCY

A condition where the veins cannot efficiently return blood to the heart, leading to fluid buildup in the legs.

- Key Features: Chronic, bilateral swelling, heaviness, aching, and varicose veins. Skin changes such as hyperpigmentation, eczema, and venous ulcers may occur.
- Risk Factors: Obesity, pregnancy, prolonged standing, history of DVT.
- Diagnostic Tests: Doppler ultrasound to assess venous flow.

5. LYMPHEDEMA

Swelling caused by impaired lymphatic drainage, often following surgery or radiation therapy that affects the lymph nodes.

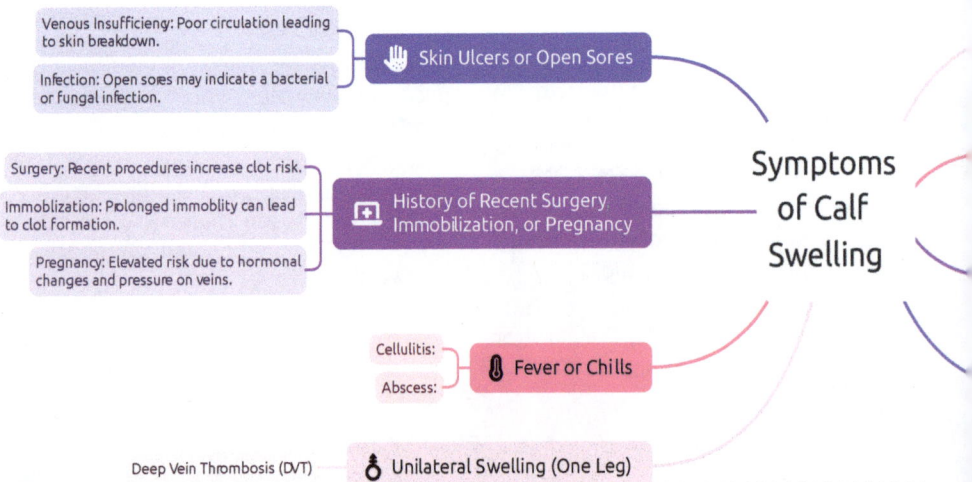

Venous Insufficieny: Poor circulation leading to skin breakdown.

Infection: Open sores may indicate a bacterial or fungal infection.

Skin Ulcers or Open Sores

Surgery: Recent procedures increase clot risk.

Immoblization: Prolonged immoblity can lead to clot formation.

Pregnancy: Elevated risk due to hormonal changes and pressure on veins.

History of Recent Surgery, Immobilization, or Pregnancy

Symptoms of Calf Swelling

Cellulitis:

Abscess:

Fever or Chills

Deep Vein Thrombosis (DVT)

Unilateral Swelling (One Leg)

- Key Features: Chronic, non-pitting oedema, often in one leg. The skin may become thickened, and there may be a sensation of heaviness or tightness.
- Risk Factors: Cancer treatment (especially lymph node dissection), infections, obesity.
- Diagnostic Tests: Clinical diagnosis, occasionally lymphoscintigraphy.

6. COMPARTMENT SYNDROME

Increased pressure within a muscle compartment that reduces blood flow and can cause muscle and nerve damage.

- Key Features: Severe pain out of proportion to injury, swelling, tightness, decreased sensation, weakness, and possible loss of pulse in the affected limb. Often follows trauma, fractures, or vigorous exercise.
- Risk Factors: Trauma, crush injuries, prolonged pressure (e.g., prolonged immobilization), exercise (e.g., exertional compartment syndrome).
- Diagnostic Tests: Clinical diagnosis with measurement of compartment pressures; MRI or ultrasound for evaluation.

7. ACHILLES TENDON RUPTURE

A rupture or tear of the Achilles tendon, typically following a sudden push-off or forceful movement.

- Key Features: Sudden pain in the calf, swelling, bruising, inability to plantarflex the foot, and difficulty walking. Often described as feeling like being "kicked" in the back of the leg.
- Risk Factors: Sports injuries (e.g., basketball, running), age-related tendon degeneration, corticosteroid use.
- Diagnostic Tests: Clinical examination (e.g., Thompson test), ultrasound, or MRI.

8. BAKER'S CYST (POPLITEAL CYST)

A fluid-filled sac that forms behind the knee, often related to joint problems such as osteoarthritis or meniscal tears.

- Key Features: Swelling in the back of the knee, tightness in the calf, and sometimes pain. The cyst may rupture, leading to calf swelling and bruising.
- Risk Factors: Knee osteoarthritis, meniscal injury, joint inflammation.
- Diagnostic Tests: Ultrasound or MRI.

9. TRAUMATIC INJURY (FRACTURE, MUSCLE TEAR, OR CONTUSION)

Trauma to the calf can result in swelling due to fractures, muscle tears, or contusions.

- Key Features: Sudden onset of swelling following trauma, localized pain, bruising, or difficulty bearing weight.
- Risk Factors: Sports injuries, falls, motor vehicle accidents, or direct trauma.

Severe Pain or Tenderness — Deep Vein Thrombosis (DVT)

Warmth and Redness
- Cellulitis
- Inflammation
- Blood Clot.

Shortness of Breath, Chest Pain, and/or Haemoptysis — Pulmonary Embolism

Sudden Onset and Rapid Progression — Traumatic Injury
- Muscle Tear
- Ruptured Achilles Tendon

- Diagnostic Tests: X-ray for fractures, MRI for soft tissue injuries.

10. OSTEOMYELITIS OR SEPTIC ARTHRITIS

Infection of the bone (osteomyelitis) or joint (septic arthritis), which can cause swelling in the affected leg.

- Key Features: Severe pain, swelling, redness, warmth, fever, and difficulty moving the joint or limb.
- Risk Factors: Recent surgery, trauma, intravenous drug use, diabetes, immunocompromised states.
- Diagnostic Tests: Blood cultures, MRI for osteomyelitis, joint aspiration for septic arthritis, X-rays.

11. MYOSITIS (MUSCLE INFLAMMATION)

Inflammation of the muscles, which can cause swelling, pain, and stiffness.

- Key Features: Muscle pain, weakness, and swelling. It may be associated with systemic symptoms such as fever, fatigue, or weight loss.
- Risk Factors: Autoimmune diseases (e.g., dermatomyositis, polymyositis), infections, trauma.
- Diagnostic Tests: Creatine kinase (CK) levels, muscle biopsy, MRI.

12. MEDICATIONS OR DRUG REACTIONS

Certain medications (e.g., calcium channel blockers, corticosteroids, NSAIDs) can cause fluid retention and calf swelling as a side effect.

- Key Features: Bilateral oedema, often without pain or significant redness. Other side effects may be present depending on the drug.
- Diagnostic Tests: Review of medications, and if necessary, blood tests to rule out other causes.

Top tip

Patients with multiple DVT s Should be investigated for malignancy

Acute Limb Ischemia: The 6 'P's

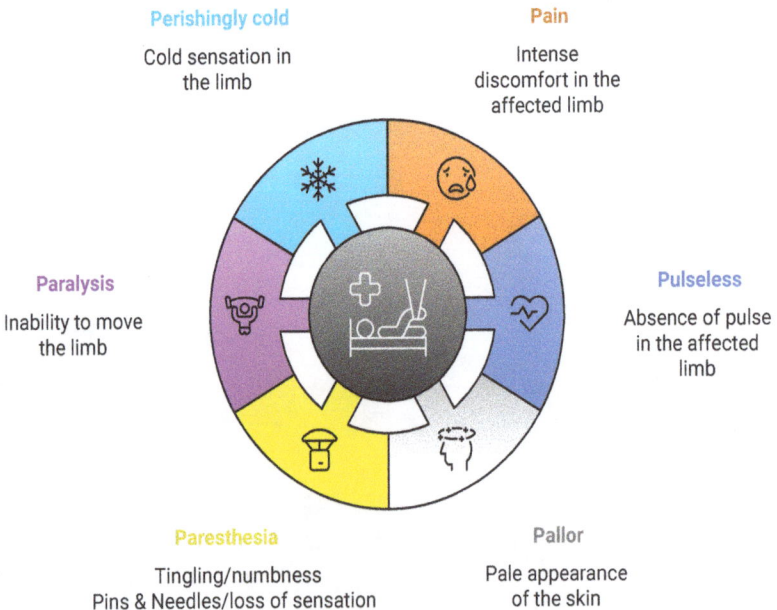

Perishingly cold
Cold sensation in the limb

Pain
Intense discomfort in the affected limb

Paralysis
Inability to move the limb

Pulseless
Absence of pulse in the affected limb

Paresthesia
Tingling/numbness Pins & Needles/loss of sensation

Pallor
Pale appearance of the skin

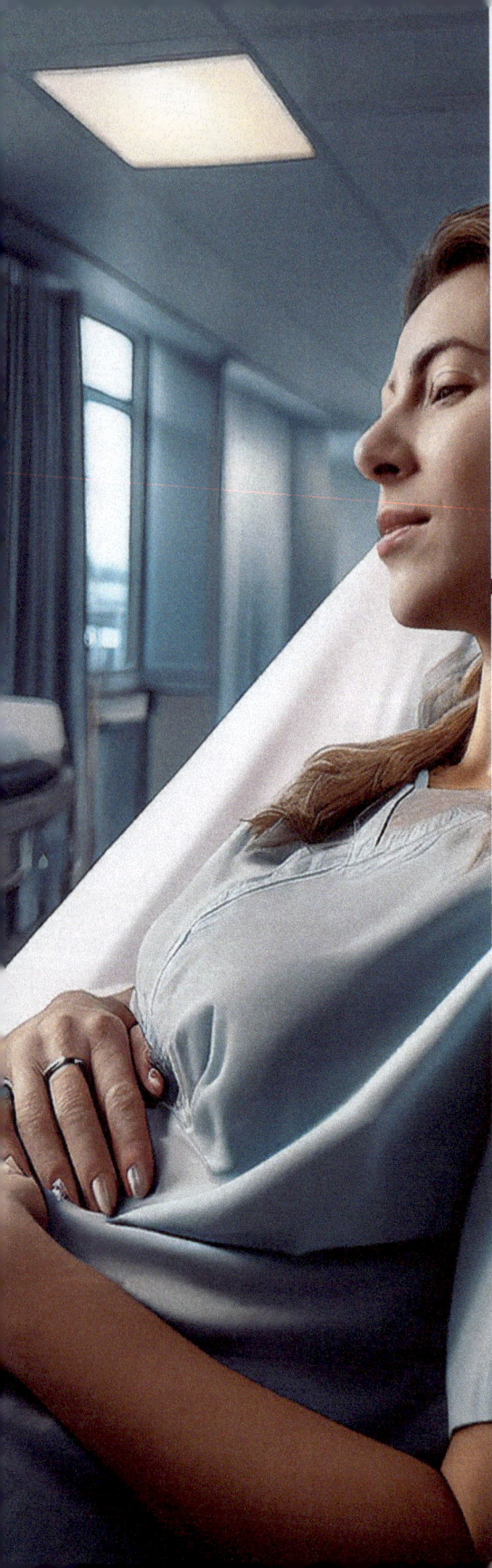

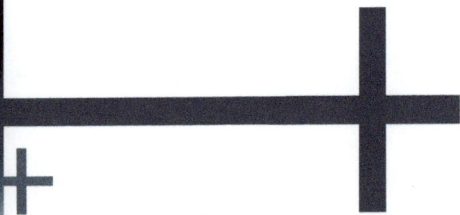

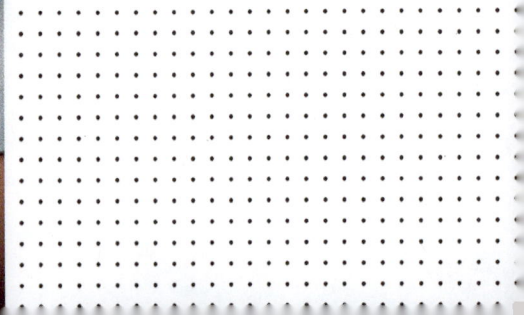

09

Abdominal Pain

Abdominal pain is interesting for its complexity and potential for life-threatening causes. Often described as the "black box" of clinical presentations*, acute abdominal pain demands a sharp diagnostic acumen and systematic evaluation. Its causes span a broad spectrum, from benign discomfort to a ruptured aortic aneurysm, necessitating a balance between urgency and precision. Accurate interpretation of signs, paired with an awareness of red flags and critical diagnoses, is vital in uncovering the underlying pathology and directing timely intervention.

*Abdominal Pain: A Black Box of Liability by Jennifer L'Hommedieu Stankus; www.acepnow.com/article/abdominal-pain-black-box-liability

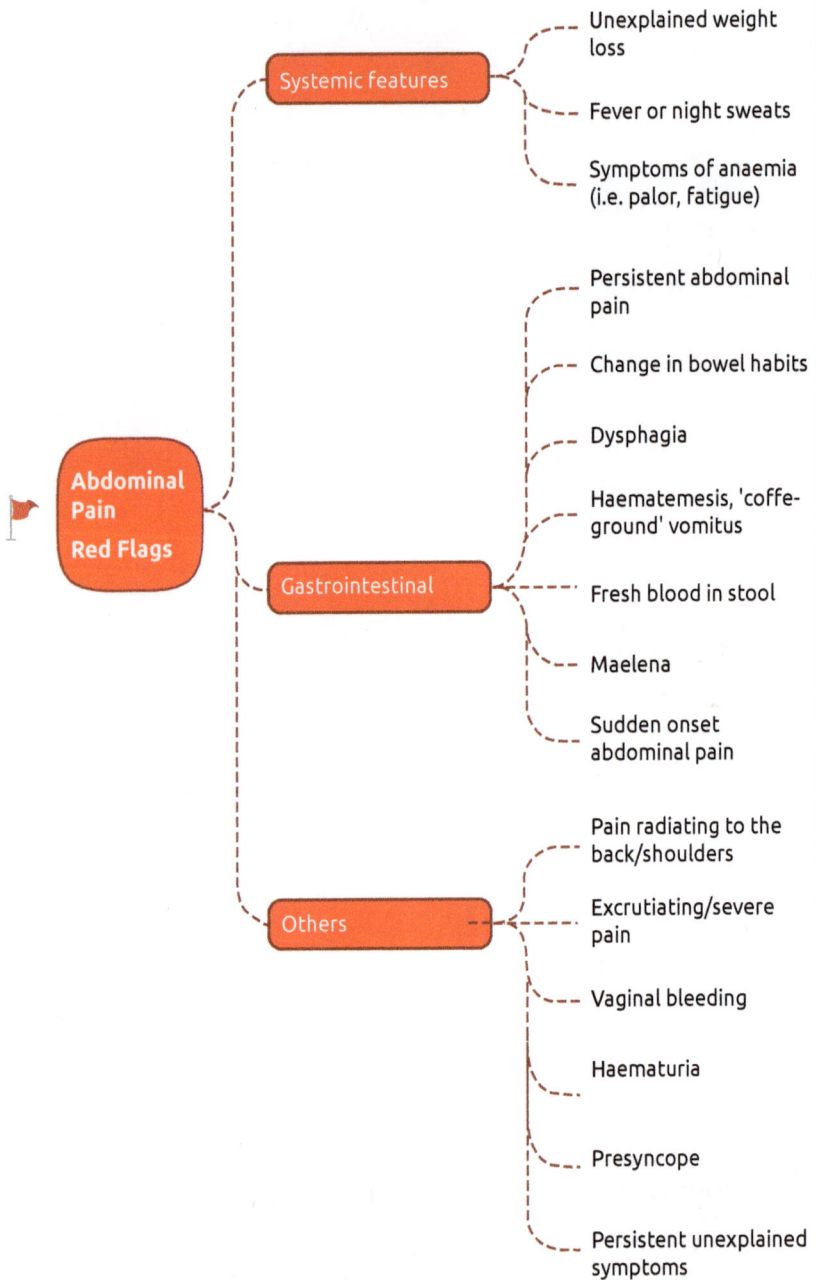

Abdominal Pain Red Flags

Systemic features
- Unexplained weight loss
- Fever or night sweats
- Symptoms of anaemia (i.e. palor, fatigue)

Gastrointestinal
- Persistent abdominal pain
- Change in bowel habits
- Dysphagia
- Haematemesis, 'coffe-ground' vomitus
- Fresh blood in stool
- Maelena
- Sudden onset abdominal pain

Others
- Pain radiating to the back/shoulders
- Excrutiating/severe pain
- Vaginal bleeding
- Haematuria
- Presyncope
- Persistent unexplained symptoms

History Taking - Important points

Where did it start?

- Location and if it has moved (e.g., RLQ migration -> appendicitis).

What were you doing when it started?

- Activity at onset (postprandial -> gallstones; exertion -> AAA rupture).

How quickly did it come on?

- Sudden onset: Renal stone, ruptured AAA, ectopic pregnancy.
- Gradual onset: Appendicitis, pancreatitis.

What is the severity and character of the pain?

- Scale 1–10; sharp, dull, crampy, or burning.
- Where is the pain now, and does it radiate?

- Back: Pancreatitis, AAA.
- Right shoulder: Gallbladder.
- Left shoulder: Spleen.
- Left arm: MI.

Associated symptoms?

- Nausea, vomiting, diarrhea, jaundice, fever, weight loss.

Does eating affect the pain?

- Relieved by eating: Duodenal ulcer.
- Worsened by eating: Gastric ulcer, biliary colic.

Is the patient pregnant?

- Always rule out ectopic pregnancy in women of childbearing age.

Are you missing something?

- **Ectopic pregnancy:** in a young female or a woman of childbearing age—always perform a pregnancy test.
- **Acute appendicitis** may masquerade as gastroenteritis.
- **Mesenteric ischemia** should be considered in elderly patients with atrial fibrillation or disproportionate pain compared to physical findings.

- **Peritonitis** often presents as severe pain with the patient lying still to minimize movement.
- **Ruptured abdominal aortic aneurysm (AAA)** presents with back pain, shock, or neurological signs.
- Vaginal bleeding or shock in a pregnant woman suggests **ruptured ectopic pregnancy.**

Top tips

CLINICAL PATTERNS TO NOTE

- Patients with biliary colic or renal colic are usually writhing in bed, trying to find a comfortable position.
- A history of previous abdominal surgery suggests the possibility of bowel obstruction due to adhesions.

APPROACH TO DIAGNOSIS

First assume the worst—rule out life-threatening conditions before exploring other diagnoses.

"5 S's"

- **S**igns of shock (e.g., hypotension, tachycardia)
- **S**igns of peritonitis (e.g., guarding, rigidity, rebound tenderness)
- **S**evere pain that is persistent or disproportionate to findings
- **S**igns of obstruction (e.g., distension, vomiting, no bowel movements)
- **S**igns of pregnancy complications (e.g., ectopic pregnancy with pain or bleeding)

Diagnostic sieves

■ □ □ +

Serious diagnoses to consider

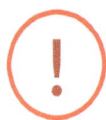

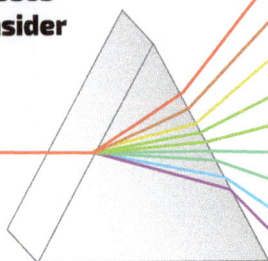

Bowel Obstruction

Abdominal Aortic Aneurysm

Perforated Viscus (e.g. from Peptic Ulcer or Diverticulitis)

Acute Pancreatitis

Mesenteric Ischaemia

Intestinal Perforation (e.g., Appendicitis, Diverticulitis)

Ectopic Pregnancy

Acute Cholecystitis or Biliary colic

Severe Gastrointestinal Bleeding

! SERIOUS SYMPTOMS!

- Sudden, severe abdominal pain: This can indicate conditions like **AAA, mesenteric ischemia, or perforation.**
- Pain radiating to the back: Often seen in **pancreatitis or AAA.**
- Nausea and vomiting: Common in **bowel obstruction, pancreatitis, and perforation.**
- Collapse, dizziness, or syncope: Suggests possible rupture (e.g., **AAA or ectopic pregnancy**) or **severe haemorrhage**
- Persistent, localized pain: Often associated with **appendicitis, cholecystitis, or diverticulitis.**
- Pain that worsens with movement or coughing: Indicates **peritoneal irritation, as in perforation or appendicitis**

! SERIOUS SIGNS!

- Hypotension, tachycardia) may indicate haemorrhagic shock (e.g., **AAA rupture**) or **sepsis**. Also pallor, diaphoresis are suggest shock or pain.
- Rigid or distended abdomen seen in **perforation, peritonitis, and advanced bowel obstruction.**
- Rebound tenderness & guarding: Signs of peritoneal irritation (**inflammation or perforation**).
- Absent/abnormal bowel sounds: May suggest **bowel obstruction or ileus.**
- Pulsatile abdominal mass: A red flag for **AAA.**
- Jaundice: think liver (e.g., **cholecystitis**).
- Visible/palpable abdominal bruising: Associated with **trauma or haemorrhagic pancreatitis.**
- Blood in vomit/stool: Indicates GI bleeding

Epigastric
· Esophagitis
· Peptic ulcer
· Perforated ulcer
· Pancreatitis

Right hypochondriac
· Gallstones
· Cholangitis
· Hepatitis
· Liver abscess
· Cardiac causes
· Lung causes

Left hypochondriac
· Spleen abscess
· Acute splenomegaly
· Spleen rupture

Umbilical
· Appendicitis (early)
· Mesenteric lymphadenitis
· Meckel diverticulitis
· Lymphomas

Right lumbar
· Ureteric colic
· Pyelonephritis

Transpyloric plane

Transtubercular plane

Left lumbar
· Ureteric colic
· Pyelonephritis

Right iliac
· Appendicitis
· Crohn disease
· Cecum obstruction
· Ovarian cyst
· Ectopic pregnancy
· Hernias

Hypogastric
· Testicular torsion
· Urinary retention
· Cystitis
· Placental abruption

Left iliac
· Diverticulitis
· Ulcerative colitis
· Constipation
· Ovarian cyst
· Hernias

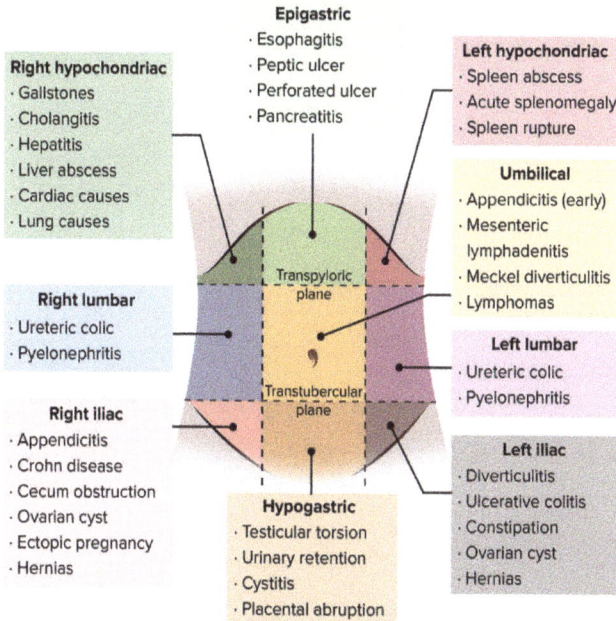

Figure 15.1
(Left) Differential diagnoses of abdominal pain by site
Courtesy lecturio.com/concepts/ acute-abdomen (Lecturio.com)

Bottom:
Differential diagnoses of abdominal pain by site

Category	Examples
V – Vascular	Ruptured abdominal aortic aneurysm (AAA), mesenteric ischemia (acute or chronic), dissection of the abdominal aorta, portal vein thrombosis, splenic infarction, myocardial infarction (referred pain).
I – Infectious	Gastroenteritis, appendicitis, diverticulitis, cholecystitis, hepatitis, pancreatitis, pyelonephritis or renal abscess, pelvic inflammatory disease, tuberculosis (abdominal), liver abscess.
T – Trauma	Blunt abdominal trauma (organ rupture: liver, spleen, bowel), penetrating injuries (knife, gunshot, or post-surgical), post-surgical adhesions causing bowel obstruction, hernia strangulation or incarceration.
A – Autoimmune	Inflammatory bowel disease (IBD) (Crohn's disease, ulcerative colitis), celiac disease, autoimmune hepatitis, systemic lupus erythematosus (SLE) with abdominal vasculitis, vasculitis (e.g., polyarteritis nodosa, Henoch-Schönlein purpura).
M – Metabolic	Diabetic ketoacidosis (DKA), hypercalcemia (e.g., from malignancy, hyperparathyroidism), hypokalemia or hyperkalemia, porphyria, adrenal insufficiency (Addisonian crisis), uraemia (chronic kidney disease-related abdominal pain), sickle cell crisis.
I – Idiopathic	Functional abdominal pain, irritable bowel syndrome (IBS), non-ulcer dyspepsia, abdominal migraine.
N – Neoplastic	Colorectal cancer, gastric cancer, hepatocellular carcinoma, pancreatic cancer, ovarian cancer, lymphoma, peritoneal carcinomatosis.
D – Degenerative	Chronic mesenteric ischemia (intestinal angina), diverticulosis, degenerative spinal disease causing referred pain.
C – Congenital	Meckel's diverticulum, congenital malrotation of the intestines, hernias (inguinal, umbilical, diaphragmatic), congenital bile duct anomalies.

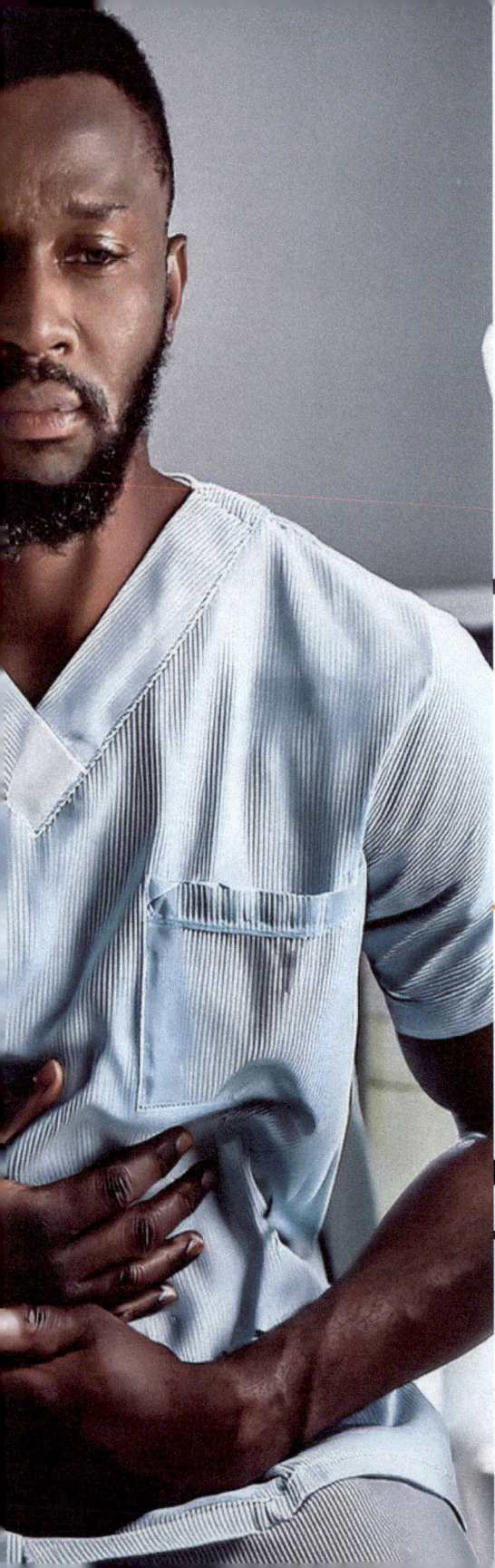

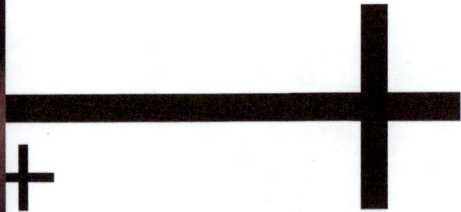

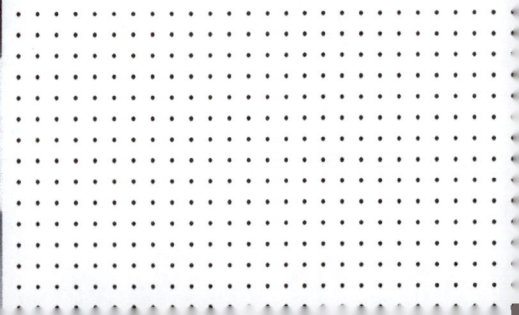

10
Constipation

Constipation is a common gastrointestinal complaint characterized by infrequent, difficult, or incomplete bowel movements. While often of benign origin (such as dietary changes or medications), it can indicate serious underlying conditions (i.e. bowel obstruction, malignancy, or neurological disorders). A structured approach to history, examination, and investigations is essential to identify red flags and differentiate functional constipation from organic causes. Timely recognition of critical diagnoses can prevent severe complications and guide effective management.

Diagnostic sieves

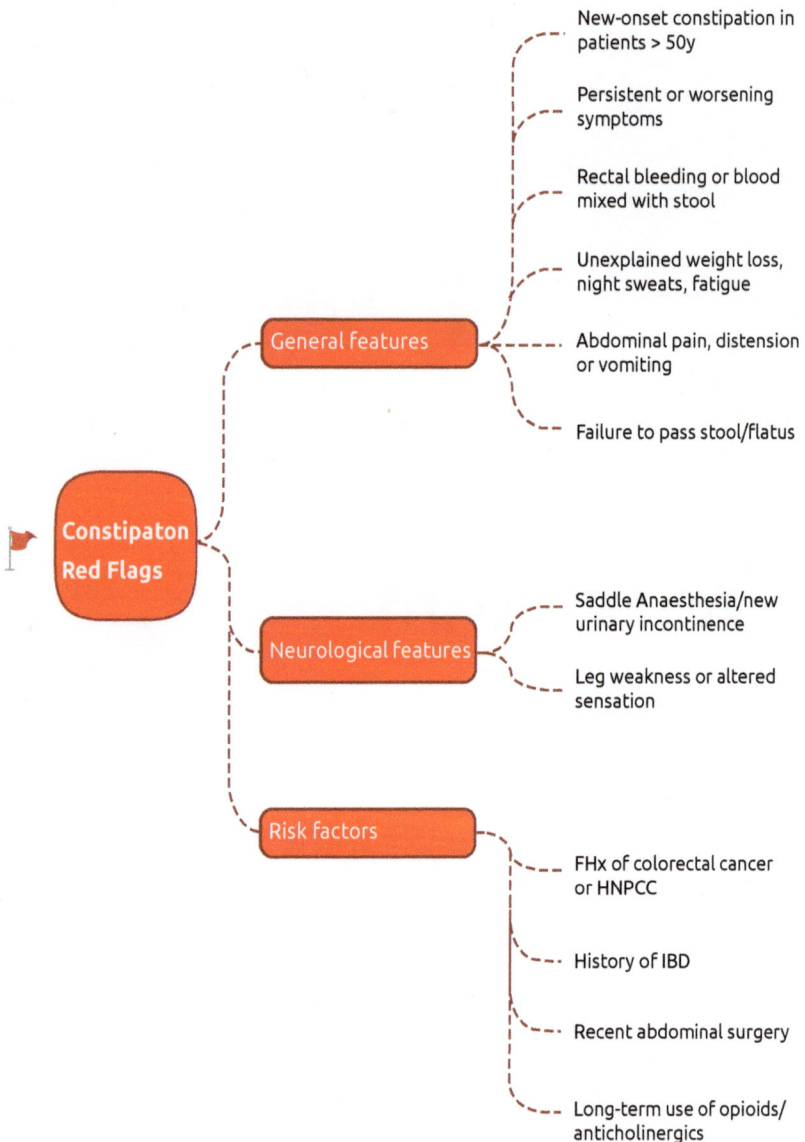

Constipaton Red Flags

General features
- New-onset constipation in patients > 50y
- Persistent or worsening symptoms
- Rectal bleeding or blood mixed with stool
- Unexplained weight loss, night sweats, fatigue
- Abdominal pain, distension or vomiting
- Failure to pass stool/flatus

Neurological features
- Saddle Anaesthesia/new urinary incontinence
- Leg weakness or altered sensation

Risk factors
- FHx of colorectal cancer or HNPCC
- History of IBD
- Recent abdominal surgery
- Long-term use of opioids/anticholinergics

History Taking - Important points

1. DURATION:
- How long has the constipation been present? Persistent constipation in older adults is concerning.

2. ABDOMINAL PAIN:
- Is there cramping, severe, or localized pain? Obstruction or IBD may be suspected.

3. BOWEL MOVEMENTS:
- Can the patient pass wind, or is there complete cessation of stool and gas? Suggests bowel obstruction.

4. BLEEDING:
- Is blood mixed with stool or streaked on the outside? Mixed suggests colorectal cancer; streaked suggests an anal disorder.

5. ALTERNATING SYMPTOMS:
- Any episodes of diarrhoea alternating with constipation? May indicate IBS, obstruction, or malignancy.

6. SYSTEMIC SYMPTOMS:
- Is there weight loss, fatigue, or night sweats? Suggest malignancy or systemic disease.

7. NEUROLOGICAL SYMPTOMS:
- Are there leg weakness, urinary issues, or saddle anaesthesia? Indicates possible cord compression.

8. MEDICAL HISTORY:
- Any history of diabetes, hypothyroidism, or abdominal surgery? Autonomic neuropathy, strictures, or adhesions could be the cause.

9. DIETARY AND LIFESTYLE:
- Has there been a recent change in diet, fluid intake, or activity level? Common factors in functional constipation.

10. STRESS:
- Is there a history of significant stress or anxiety? Could indicate IBS.

11. MEDICATIONS:
- Are they using opioids, anticholinergics, or other constipating drugs?

Are you missing something?

- Always rule out obstruction before labelling constipation as functional.
- Constipation with weight loss or rectal bleeding is colorectal cancer until proven otherwise.
- Persistent constipation in patients <25 years warrants further investigation for organic pathology.

Clinical Patterns to Note

- Chronic use of opioids or anticholinergics often causes constipation.
- Alternating constipation and diarrhoea with abdominal pain may indicate IBS or malignancy.
- Consider hypercalcemia in patients with constipation and systemic symptoms (e.g., polyuria, bone pain).

Top tips

APPROACH TO DIAGNOSIS

Perform a thorough abdominal and rectal examination, including digital rectal exam for faecal impaction or masses.

Order blood tests (FBC, TSH, calcium, glucose) and imaging (e.g., abdominal X-ray) when red flags are present.

Use criteria such as Rome IV for diagnosing

Serious diagnoses to consider

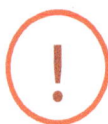

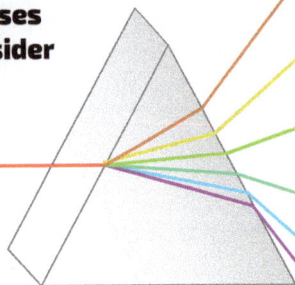

Colorectal Cancer

Bowel Obstruction

Cauda Equina Syndrome

IBD

Hypercalcemia (e.g. Parathyroid Adenoma, Malignancy-related)

Autonomic Neuropathy (e.g. Diabetes-related)

! SERIOUS SYMPTOMS!

- Constipation with rectal bleeding or weight loss: Suggests **malignancy or advanced IBD.**
- Alternating constipation and diarrhea: May indicate **colorectal cancer, IBS, or partial obstruction.**
- Severe abdominal pain and failure to pass gas: **Bowel obstruction likely.**
- Numbness, weakness, or incontinence with constipation: Suggestive of **spinal cord compression or cauda equina syndrome.**

! SERIOUS SIGNS!

- Palpable abdominal or rectal mass: Indicates **malignancy or fecal impaction.**
- Abdominal distension with tympany on percussion: Suggests **bowel obstruction.**
- Hyperreflexia or reduced anal tone: May indicate **neurological causes (e.g., spinal cord lesion).**
- Dry mucous membranes or other signs of dehydration: May indicate severe systemic illness.

functional constipation or IBS.

Refer for colonoscopy in patients with persistent symptoms, red flags, or family history of colorectal cancer.

Differential diagnoses of constipation using the VITAMIN DC framework

Category	Examples
V – Vascular	Mesenteric ischemia or infarction, chronic mesenteric ischemia.
I – Infectious	Infectious colitis (e.g., *Clostridium difficile*, tuberculosis), parasitic infections (e.g., *Strongyloides*, *Schistosomiasis*), rectal or perianal abscess or fistula causing obstruction.
T – Traumatic	Post-surgical adhesions, pelvic or spinal trauma leading to nerve or bowel dysfunction.
A – Autoimmune	Crohn's disease with strictures, ulcerative colitis with stenosis, systemic sclerosis.
M – Metabolic/Endocrine	Hypothyroidism, hypercalcemia (e.g., hyperparathyroidism, malignancy), diabetes mellitus causing autonomic neuropathy, hypokalemia or hypermagnesemia, adrenal insufficiency, porphyria presenting with episodic constipation.
I – Idiopathic/Functional	Chronic idiopathic constipation, irritable bowel syndrome with constipation (IBS-C), psychological conditions (e.g., depression or eating disorders).
N – Neoplastic	Colorectal cancer or rectal cancer, pelvic malignancies (e.g., ovarian, uterine cancers causing mass effect).
D – Degenerative/Neurological	Spinal cord lesions (e.g., cauda equina syndrome, multiple sclerosis), Parkinson's disease with gastrointestinal dysmotility.
C – Congenital	Hirschsprung's disease (congenital aganglionic megacolon, may present late in adults), intestinal malrotation or other anatomical abnormalities.

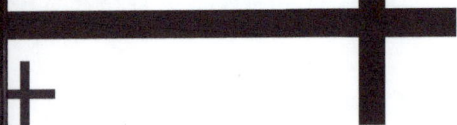

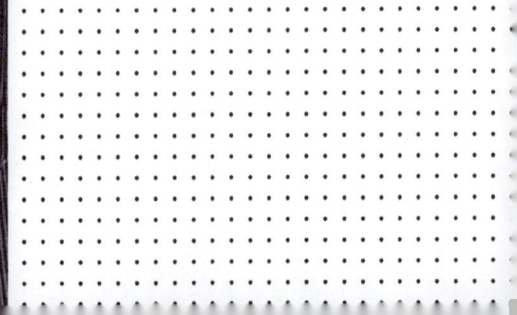

11

Jaundice

■ **Jaundice** refers to the yellow discoloration of the skin, sclerae, and mucous membranes caused by elevated serum bilirubin levels (>2 mg/dL or 34 µmol/L). It results from an imbalance in bilirubin production and clearance. Jaundice is often classified into three categories based on pathophysiology: pre-hepatic (hemolysis or ineffective erythropoiesis), hepatic (liver dysfunction), and post-hepatic (biliary obstruction). Identifying the underlying cause is crucial to guide management.

Jaundice Red Flags

- Painless jaundice in older adults
- Fever and RUQ pain
- Confusion, altered mental state
- Severe abdominal pain radiating to the back
- Rapidly worsening jaundice, coagulopathy
- Systemic signs (fever, rash, joint pain)
- Unexplained weight loss or night sweats

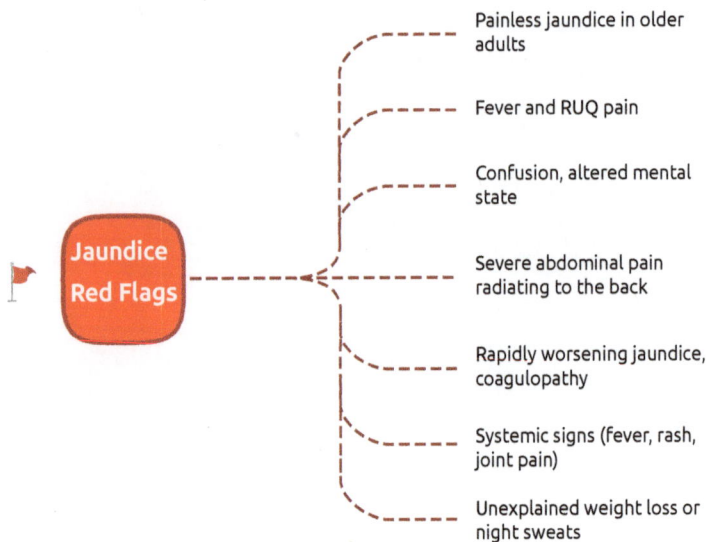

Differential diagnoses of jaundice using the VITAMIN CDE framework

Category	Examples
V – Vascular	Ischemic hepatitis, Budd-Chiari syndrome.
I – Infectious	Viral hepatitis (A, B, C, E), leptospirosis, malaria, sepsis.
T – Toxicological	Alcohol-related liver disease, paracetamol overdose, amanita mushroom poisoning.
A – Autoimmune	Autoimmune hepatitis, primary biliary cholangitis (PBC), primary sclerosing cholangitis (PSC).
M – Metabolic	Hemochromatosis, Wilson's disease, alpha-1 antitrypsin deficiency.
I – Idiopathic	Gilbert syndrome, Crigler-Najjar syndrome.
N – Neoplastic	Pancreatic cancer, cholangiocarcinoma, hepatocellular carcinoma.
C – Congenital	Biliary atresia, choledochal cysts.
D – Degenerative	End-stage liver disease.
E – Environmental	Aflatoxin exposure, industrial chemical exposure.

History Taking

1. ONSET:

What is the duration of jaundice?

- Insidious onset over several weeks suggests malignancy, especially in older patients.
- Acute onset raises suspicion of cholangitis or viral hepatitis.

2. RISK FACTORS:

- Recent travel (e.g., regions endemic for hepatitis).
- Blood transfusions, IV drug use, or risky sexual behavior (risk for hepatitis B or C).
- History of previous jaundice, chronic liver disease, gallstones, or alcohol excess.
- Family history of liver disease (e.g., Wilson's, Gilbert syndrome).

3. ASSOCIATED SYMPTOMS:

- Fever, joint pains, and rash before jaundice: Suggest hepatitis B.

- Fever and rigors: Suggest acute cholangitis.
- Weight loss and back pain: Suggest malignancy.
- Features of chronic liver disease: Such as ascites.
- Epigastric pain: Suggest pancreatitis or pancreatic cancer.
- Pruritus: Suggests a cholestatic process.

4. OTHER SPECIFIC FEATURES:

- Exposure to someone with hepatitis.
- History of pruritus or arthritis: Suggests hemochromatosis.
- Worsening jaundice with viral illness: Points to Gilbert syndrome.
- Epigastric pain with pale stools and dark urine: Suggests biliary obstruction.

Common causes of jaundice:

Pre-hepatic jaundice	Hepatic	Post-hepatic jaundice
Hemolysis - hereditary spherocytosis, sickle cell disease, G6PD deficiency *Ineffective erythropoiesis* - like thalassemia, megaloblastic anemia *Hematoma resorption* *Gilbert syndrome* *Crigler-Najjar syndrome (Type I and II)*	*Viral hepatitis* *Alcoholic hepatitis* *Autoimmune hepatitis* *Drug-induced liver injury* *Cirrhosis* - ie. alcoholic, non-alcoholic steatohepatitis, viral, autoimmune *Hemochromatosis* *Wilson's disease* *Alpha-1 antitrypsin deficiency* *Leptospirosis* *Sepsis-related cholestasis.* *Ischemic hepatitis (shock liver)*	*Gallstones (choledocho-lithiasis)* *Biliary strictures* *Pancreatic cancer* *Cholangiocarcinoma* *Primary sclerosing cholangitis (PSC)* *Biliary atresia* *Parasites (ie. liver flukes)* *Post-operative biliary injury* *Mirizzi syndrome*

Diagnostic sieves

Serious diagnoses to consider

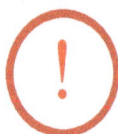

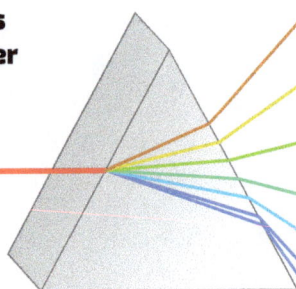

Acute Liver Failure

Cholangitis

Pancreatic Cancer

Chronic Liver Disease

Viral Hepatitis

Biliary Obstruction

Haemolysis

⚠ SERIOUS SYMPTOMS!

- Rapidly worsening jaundice: Suggests **acute liver failure or malignancy.**
- Severe abdominal pain radiating to the back: Points to **pancreatitis or pancreatic cancer.**
- Fever with jaundice: Suggests **cholangitis or viral hepatitis.**
- Weight loss and night sweats: Red flags for **malignancy or TB.**
- Bleeding tendency and confusion: Indicates **hepatic encephalopathy and coagulopathy**

⚠ SERIOUS SIGNS!

- Jaundice with fever and RUQ tenderness: Suggests **cholangitis.**
- Stigmata of chronic liver disease: Includes **ascites, spider naevi, and palmar erythema.**
- Distended abdomen with tenderness: Indicates **severe ascites or peritonitis.**
- Pallor with jaundice: Suggests **hemolysis or severe anemia.**
- Dark urine and pale stools: Indicative of **biliary obstruction.**
- Hypotension or tachycardia: Suggests **sepsis or significant hypovolemia**

Serious diagnoses to consider

1. ACUTE LIVER FAILURE:

Rapid onset jaundice, encephalopathy, coagulopathy. Diagnostic tools: INR > 1.5, elevated transaminases, ammonia levels.

2. CHOLANGITIS:

Charcot's triad (jaundice, fever, RUQ pain) or Reynold's pentad (adds shock and altered mental status). Diagnostic tools: LFTs, blood cultures, ultrasound/MRCP.

3. PANCREATIC CANCER:

Painless jaundice, weight loss, back pain. Diagnostic tools: CT abdomen, CA 19-9.

4. CHRONIC LIVER DISEASE:

Stigmata of liver disease (spider naevi, ascites, palmar erythema). Diagnostic tools: LFTs, ultrasound with elastography.

5. VIRAL HEPATITIS:

Fever, fatigue, dark urine, anorexia. Diagnostic tools: Viral serology (Hepatitis A, B, C).

6. BILIARY OBSTRUCTION:

Intermittent RUQ pain, pale stools, dark urine. Diagnostic tools: Abdominal ultrasound, MRCP.

7. HAEMOLYSIS:

Pallor, dark urine, splenomegaly. Diagnostic tools: Blood smear, LDH, haptoglobin, reticulocyte count.

Diagnostic approach

Initial Tests:

- LFTs: Bilirubin, ALT, AST, ALP, GGT.
  Approach to deranged LFTs:
  Do they have liver disease?
  What type of liver disease?
  How severe is it?
  Stage of disease?
  How much liver fibrosis?
      - *Consider Fib4 score, iLFTs.*

FIB-4 score is a non-invasive index used to estimate the amount of liver fibrosis & need for biopsy in patients with chronic liver disease. iLFTs enhance the accuracy and efficiency of diagnosing liver disease.

- Full blood count: Hemolysis or infection.

- Coagulation profile: Assess INR.
- Viral serology: Hepatitis A, B, C, and E.

Imaging:

- Abdominal Ultrasound: First-line for biliary obstruction.
- MRCP or CT Scan: For further evaluation of obstruction or malignancy.

Specialist Tests:

- Autoimmune Markers: ANA, AMA, ASMA for autoimmune hepatitis or PBC.
- Tumor Markers: CA 19-9, AFP for pancreatic or hepatocellular carcinoma.

Liver Biopsy:

- For unexplained hepatic jaundice or suspected autoimmune conditions.

When to admit

Acute Liver Failure:

- Jaundice with encephalopathy or coagulopathy.
- Severe acidosis (pH < 7.3), bilirubin >300 µmol/L.

Cholangitis:

- Charcot's triad with sepsis or shock.

- Requires IV antibiotics and urgent ERCP.

Rapidly Worsening Jaundice:

- Suggesting fulminant liver failure or malignancy.

CONSIDER HEPATOLOGY REFERRAL IF:

• All liver screen tests negative/normal but ALT persistently raised > twice ULN or AST>ALT

• HBsAg or HCV Ab positive(even if LFTs have normalised)

• Any liver auto-antibodies positive

• Ferritin > 500

• USS features of cirrhosis &/or portal hypertension (ascites, big spleen, low platelets).

• USS shows liver lesions.

Abnormal Aminotransferase Values of Unknown Cause: Proposed Algorithm for Primary Care Management/Referral to Hepatology Services. Dr SA Khan, Dr J Fluxman, Prof M Thursz

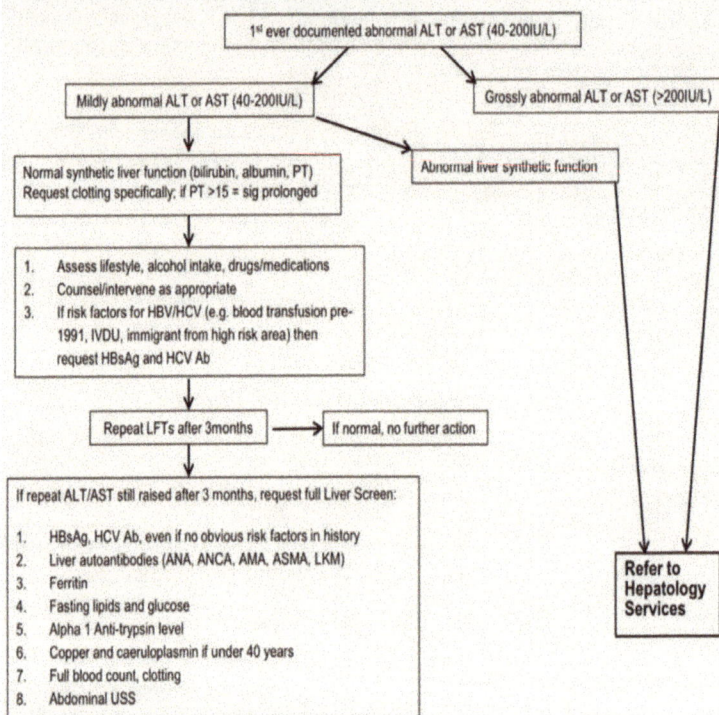

1st ever documented abnormal ALT or AST (40-200IU/L)

Mildly abnormal ALT or AST (40-200IU/L)

Grossly abnormal ALT or AST (>200IU/L)

Normal synthetic liver function (bilirubin, albumin, PT) Request clotting specifically: if PT >15 = sig prolonged

Abnormal liver synthetic function

1. Assess lifestyle, alcohol intake, drugs/medications
2. Counsel/intervene as appropriate
3. If risk factors for HBV/HCV (e.g. blood transfusion pre-1991, IVDU, immigrant from high risk area) then request HBsAg and HCV Ab

Repeat LFTs after 3months → If normal, no further action

If repeat ALT/AST still raised after 3 months, request full Liver Screen:

1. HBsAg, HCV Ab, even if no obvious risk factors in history
2. Liver autoantibodies (ANA, ANCA, AMA, ASMA, LKM)
3. Ferritin
4. Fasting lipids and glucose
5. Alpha 1 Anti-trypsin level
6. Copper and caeruloplasmin if under 40 years
7. Full blood count, clotting
8. Abdominal USS

Refer to Hepatology Services

Courtesy Dr S A Khan Consultant hepatologist

Mneumonic for causes of acute liver failure

TABOO

Toxins : Drugs, Alcohols, Herbal

Autoimmune hepatitis

hepatitis **B** and other infections

Occlusion of the Hepatic vein (Thrombosis, Ischaemic hepatitis)

Obstetric causes (Acute fatty liver of Pregnancy, HELLP)

Oncologic

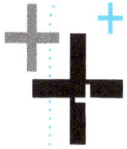

Cerebral oedema

Hypoglycaemia

Cardiac Failure

ARDS

Coagulopathy

Hypoadrenalism

AKI

Upper GI Bleed

Pancreatitis

Infections

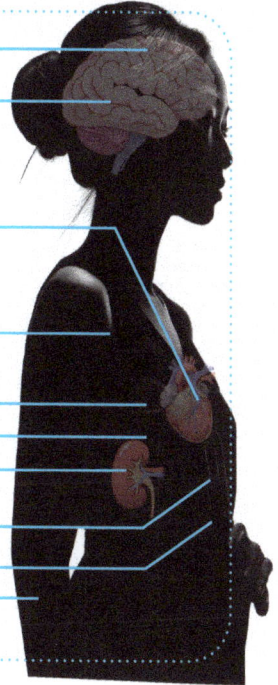

Complications of Acute Liver Failure

Are you missing somthing?

I. ACUTE LIVER FAILURE

Also known as fulminant hepatic failure

Defined as : (in a patient with no known Liver disease)

- Coagulopathy abnormality (INR> 1.5) and
- Mental alteration (hepatic encephalopathy) and
- Duration of > 8 weeks

Clinical features: Jaundice, encephalopathy, coagulopathy, abnormal LFT, ascites.

Decompensation of Chronic liver disease may be precipitated by: Dehydration, Constipation , drugs (opioids)

, alcohol

infections, GI bleed, renal failure, non compliance with treatment

Investigation: FBC, UEC, Coagulation profile, LFT, CRP, Paracetamol level, Ammonia level, USS Liver, ECG

Refer to Liver unit if:

- Acidotic (PH < 7.3)
- High lactate (> 3)

- INR > 1.5
- Bilirubin > 300 umol/L
- Hepatic encephalopathy

2. HEPATIC ENCEPHALOPATHY

This is defined as brain dysfunction caused by Liver insufficiency and/or Porto- systemic Shunting

West Haven Classification Grade Description

- Personality changes
- Personality changes, Lethargy, Asterix is Disorientated for time
- Bizarre behaviour Disorientated for time a piece Reduced consciousness
- Comatose

Clinical features: Mild to moderate symptoms of HE may include mental and physical changes:

- Mental: Mild confusion, short attention span, forgetfulness, mood swings, personality changes, inappropriate behaviour, difficulty doing basic math.
- Physical: Change in sleep patterns (like

sleeping during the day and staying up at night), difficulty writing or doing other small hand movements, breath that smells musty or sweet, slurred speech.

More severe symptoms may include:

- Mental: Marked confusion, severe anxiety or fearfulness, disorientation regarding time and place, inability to perform mental tasks such as doing basic math.
- Physical: Extreme sleepiness, slowed or sluggish movement, shaking of hands or arms (called "flapping"), jumbled, slurred speech that can't be understood.

In the most severe form of HE, patients can become unresponsive, unconscious and enter a coma.

Common precipitants: Acute kidney injury, electrolyte imbalance, gastrointestinal bleeding, infection, constipation, sedative drugs (eg, opiates, benzodiazepines, antidepressants and antipsychotic drugs), diuretics, high protein intake.

3. SPONTANEOUS BACTERIAL PERITO-NITIS

SBP is defined as a neutrophil count > 250 mm Hg in ascitic fluid

Clinical features: Abdominal pain, diarrhoea and vomiting, illeus, sepsis, shock, renal failure, worsening renal function. Can also be asymptomatic. Carries in hospital mortality of 30 percent.

4. ACUTE CHOLANGITIS

Biliary obstruction leading to infection proximal to the Obstruction. Should be

Assessment and management

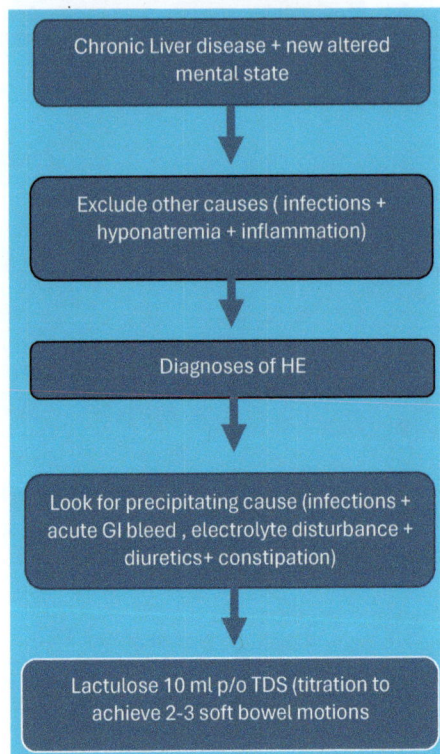

```
┌─────────────────────────────────┐
│  Chronic Liver disease + new altered │
│         mental state             │
└─────────────────────────────────┘
                │
                ▼
┌─────────────────────────────────┐
│  Exclude other causes ( infections + │
│    hyponatremia + inflammation)  │
└─────────────────────────────────┘
                │
                ▼
┌─────────────────────────────────┐
│        Diagnoses of HE           │
└─────────────────────────────────┘
                │
                ▼
┌─────────────────────────────────┐
│ Look for precipitating cause (infections + │
│ acute GI bleed , electrolyte disturbance + │
│      diuretics+ constipation)    │
└─────────────────────────────────┘
                │
                ▼
┌─────────────────────────────────┐
│ Lactulose 10 ml p/o TDS (titration to │
│  achieve 2-3 soft bowel motions  │
└─────────────────────────────────┘
```

suspected in a febrile jaundice Patient

Aetiologies: CBD Stone, stricture, malignancy.

Clinical features:

- Charcot's triad: RUQ Pain, Jaundice, fever/chills
- Sepsis
- Shock

Top Tips

- Painless jaundice in older adults is pancreatic cancer until proven otherwise.
- Always rule out hepatitis in acute jaundice cases with systemic symptoms.
- Consider autoimmune causes in younger patients with persistent jaundice.
- Assess INR and encephalopathy for signs of acute liver failure.

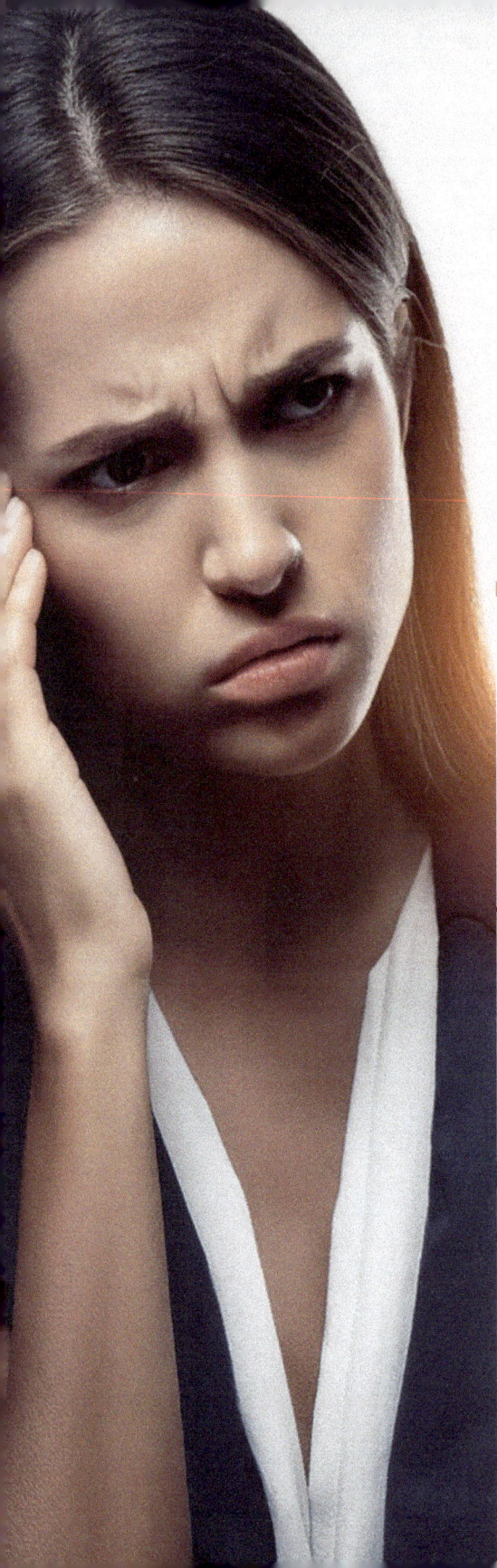

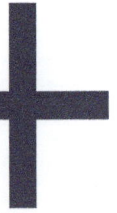

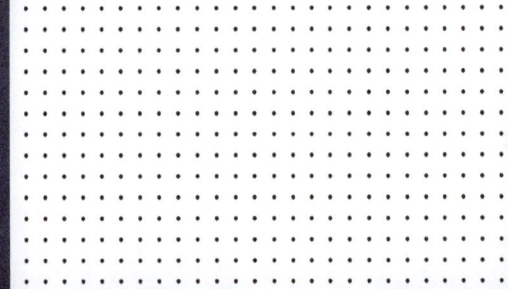

12

Diarrhoea

- **Diarrhoea** is defined as the passage of loose or watery stools, typically occurring three or more times per day. It can range from an acute, self-limiting condition caused by infections to a chronic symptom of underlying systemic or gastrointestinal disease. Accurate evaluation involves distinguishing between acute and chronic diarrhoea and identifying red flags that may indicate serious conditions such as inflammatory bowel disease (IBD), malignancy, or infection. A structured approach to history, examination, and targeted investigations ensures effective management.

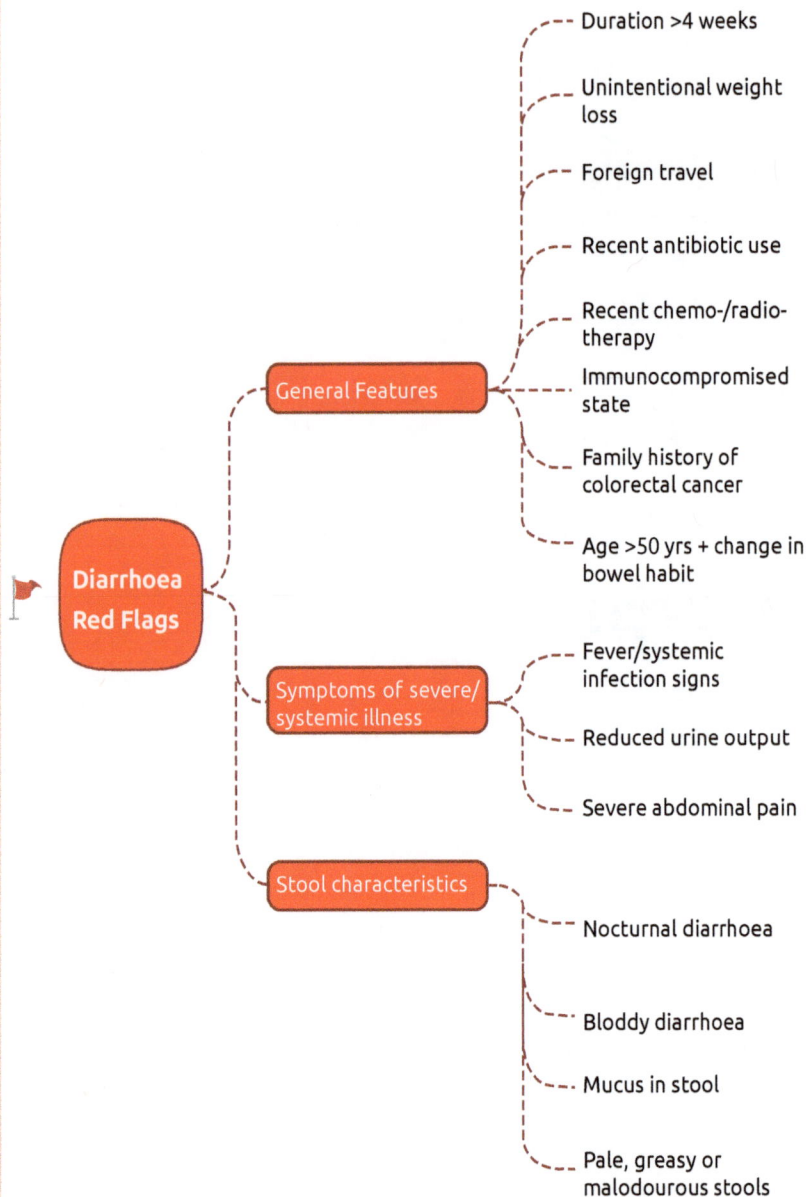

Diarrhoea Red Flags

General Features
- Duration >4 weeks
- Unintentional weight loss
- Foreign travel
- Recent antibiotic use
- Recent chemo-/radio-therapy
- Immunocompromised state
- Family history of colorectal cancer
- Age >50 yrs + change in bowel habit

Symptoms of severe/systemic illness
- Fever/systemic infection signs
- Reduced urine output
- Severe abdominal pain

Stool characteristics
- Nocturnal diarrhoea
- Bloddy diarrhoea
- Mucus in stool
- Pale, greasy or malodourous stools

History Taking - Important points

1. DURATION OF SYMPTOMS
- Short history: Likely infectious cause.
- Chronic in older patients: Consider malignancy.
- Recurrent with blood, weight loss, and systemic upset: Suggests IBD.

2. PRECIPITATING FACTORS
Use of new medications?
  i. Laxatives, antibiotics (C. difficile infection).

Recent travel?
  i. Tropical infections or parasites.

Dietary changes?
  i. Intolerances.

3. NATURE OF THE DIARRHOEA
- Bloody stools: Suggests colonic pathology (IBD, ischaemic colitis, malignancy).
- Large volume watery stools: Suggests small bowel involvement.
- Bulky, offensive stools difficult to flush: Indicates malabsorption (e.g., coeliac).
- Nocturnal diarrhoea: Points to organic pathology (e.g., IBD).
- Overflow diarrhoea: Consider constipation in older adults.

4. ASSOCIATED SYMPTOMS
- Weight loss: Suggests malabsorption, IBD, or malignancy.
- Fever: Suggests infection or IBD flare.
- Abdominal pain: Sudden onset with bloody diarrhoea in an elderly patient suggests mesenteric ischaemia or ischaemic colitis.
- Faintness or postural dizziness: Indicates dehydration or fluid depletion.
- Faeculent vomiting: Suggests bowel obstruction.
- Flushing or wheezing: Consider carcinoid syndrome.

5. PAST AND FAMILY HISTORY
- Personal or family history of IBD or colorectal cancer.
- History of bowel surgery: Potential bacterial overgrowth or altered transit time.
- History of laxative abuse or eating disorder?

6. KEY RED FLAGS TO ELICIT
- Symptoms of bowel cancer: Blood in stools, unintentional weight loss, abdominal mass, pain on defecation, or jaundice.
- Systemic signs: Anaemia, lymphadenopathy.
- Risk factors for mesenteric ischaemia: Older age, AF, metabolic acidosis, or raised lactate on ABG.

Are you missing something?

1. MESENTERIC ISCHEMIA
- Suspect in older patients with atherosclerotic risk factors, atrial fibrillation, abdominal pain, melena, bloody diarrhoea, raised lactate, and metabolic acidosis.

2. ACUTE SEVERE COLITIS:
- Look for >10 stools/day, persistent bleeding, abdominal tenderness or distension, transfusion requirements, and colonic dilatation on AXR.

3. GASTROINTESTINAL BLEED (MASSIVE):
- Presents with melena, tachycardia, hypotension, bloody diarrhoea, history of peptic ulcer disease or chronic liver disease.

4. ADDISONIAN CRISIS:
- Suspect with hypotension, diarrhoea, abdominal pain, weight loss, fatigue,

Serious diagnoses to consider

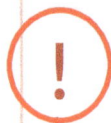

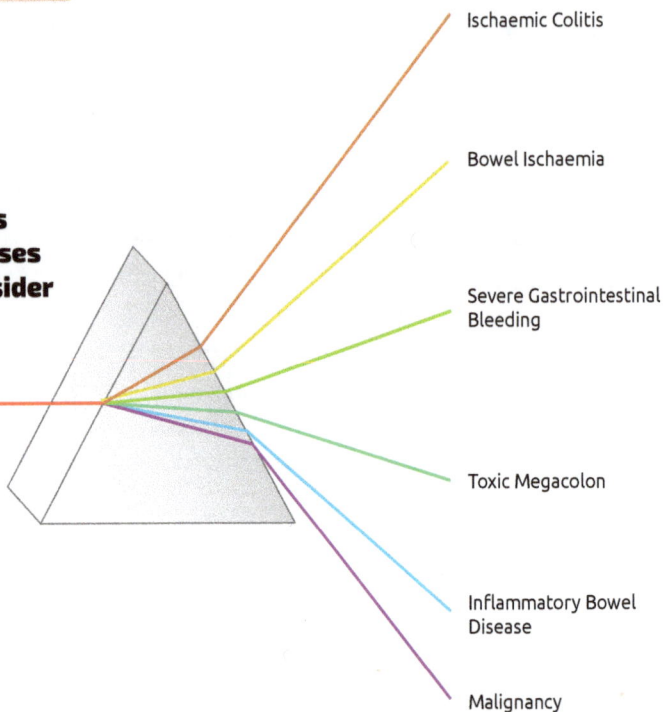

Ischaemic Colitis

Bowel Ischaemia

Severe Gastrointestinal Bleeding

Toxic Megacolon

Inflammatory Bowel Disease

Malignancy

! SERIOUS SYMPTOMS!

- Severe abdominal pain: Suggests ischaemic colitis, bowel ischaemia, or perforation.
- Bloody diarrhoea: A red flag for IBD, ischaemic colitis, or malignancy.
- Unintentional weight loss: Seen in malignancy, IBD, or malabsorption syndromes.
- Persistent diarrhoea >4 weeks: Suggests a chronic cause, including IBD or malignancy.
- Fever and systemic symptoms: Seen in infections, IBD flares, or toxic megacolon.

! SERIOUS SIGNS!

- Hemodynamic instability: Hypotension and tachycardia may indicate shock due to sepsis or significant blood loss.
- Pallor and signs of anaemia: Can occur with chronic GI bleeding or IBD.
- Guarding, rebound tenderness: Indicative of peritonitis, bowel ischaemia, or perforation.
- Distended abdomen: May suggest obstruction or toxic megacolon.
- Skin findings: E.g., erythema nodosum or pyoderma gangrenosum in IBD.
- Blood in stool (melaena or haematochezia): Indicates upper or lower GI bleeding, respectively.
- Decreased urine output: A marker of severe dehydration or AKI from diarrhoea.

shock, hypoglycaemia, or increased pigmentation.

5. INFLAMMATORY BOWEL DISEASE (IBD):
- Consider if diarrhoea persists for >2 weeks with systemic upset and negative stool

cultures.

6. COLORECTAL CANCER:
- Be alert for persistent rectal bleeding, significant weight loss, or anaemia in middle-aged and elderly patients.

Top tips

1. CLINICAL PATTERNS TO NOTE
- Weight loss in chronic diarrhoea is a concerning feature for organic pathology such as malignancy or IBD.
- Most acute cases are infectious and self-limiting, but consider stool cultures if symptoms persist beyond 1 week or are severe (e.g., fever, blood in stools).
- Beware of diagnosing Irritable Bowel Syndrome (IBS) for the first time in middle-aged or elderly patients without ruling out organic causes.
- Anaemia, rectal bleeding, or nocturnal symptoms are concerning and warrant

further investigation.
- Beware of overflow diarrhoea in older patients, especially with a history of chronic constipation.

2. APPROACH TO DIAGNOSIS
- First assume the worst—rule out life-threatening conditions like mesenteric ischaemia, fulminant colitis, or GI bleed before exploring less serious causes.

3. "4 S'S" IN ACUTE DIARRHOEA:
- Signs of shock: Hypotension, tachycardia, dehydration.

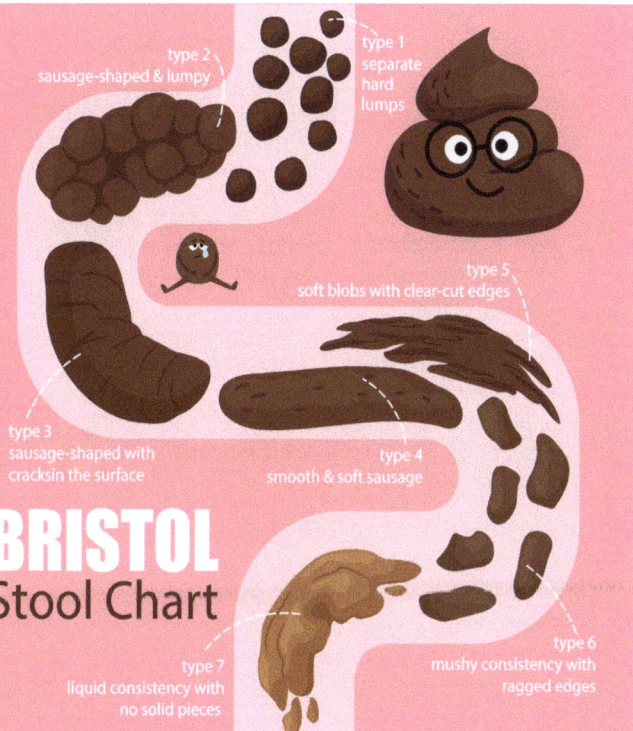

Faecal calprotectin is useful to exclude IBD and confirm IBS as a likely diagnosis when IBD is suspected but not clear.

type 2
sausage-shaped & lumpy

type 1
separate
hard
lumps

type 5
soft blobs with clear-cut edges

type 3
sausage-shaped with
cracks in the surface

type 4
smooth & soft sausage

BRISTOL
Stool Chart

type 7
liquid consistency with
no solid pieces

type 6
mushy consistency with
ragged edges

stock.adobe.com/uk/search?k=bristol+stool+chart&asset_id=634461918

Differential diagnoses of diarrhoea using the VITAMIN C framework

Category	Examples
V – Vascular	Ischaemic colitis, mesenteric ischaemia (acute or chronic), portal vein thrombosis, congestive heart failure (leading to intestinal oedema).
I – Infectious	Acute infective gastroenteritis: Bacterial (Salmonella, Shigella, Campylobacter, Clostridium difficile), Viral (Norovirus, Rotavirus), Parasitic (Giardia lamblia, Entamoeba histolytica). Abdominal tuberculosis, HIV-related infections, helminthic infestations (e.g., Strongyloides, Ascaris).
T – Trauma	Post-radiation enteritis, trauma-induced bowel injury leading to malabsorption.
A – Autoimmune	Inflammatory bowel disease (Crohn's disease, ulcerative colitis), coeliac disease, microscopic colitis (lymphocytic, collagenous), systemic lupus erythematosus (SLE) with bowel involvement.
M – Metabolic	Thyrotoxicosis, adrenal insufficiency, diabetic autonomic neuropathy, hypercalcaemia, lactose intolerance, bile acid malabsorption.
I – Idiopathic	Irritable bowel syndrome (IBS), functional diarrhoea, non-coeliac gluten sensitivity.
N – Neoplastic	Colorectal cancer, lymphoma, pancreatic cancer (malabsorption due to pancreatic insufficiency), carcinoid syndrome (associated with flushing and secretory diarrhoea).
C – Congenital	Meckel's diverticulum, congenital enzyme deficiencies (e.g., lactase deficiency).

- Severe symptoms: Persistent or disproportionate pain, frequent stools (>10/day), nocturnal diarrhoea.
- Signs of obstruction or perforation: Abdominal distension, rebound tenderness, guarding.
- Significant red flags: Weight loss, rectal bleeding, anaemia, or continuous symptoms >3 months.

Use **faecal calprotectin** to confirm IBS if IBD is suspected but not clear.

Avoid repeated stool tests if the first is negative unless there's a strong clinical indication (e.g., immunocompromised patients or persistent symptoms).

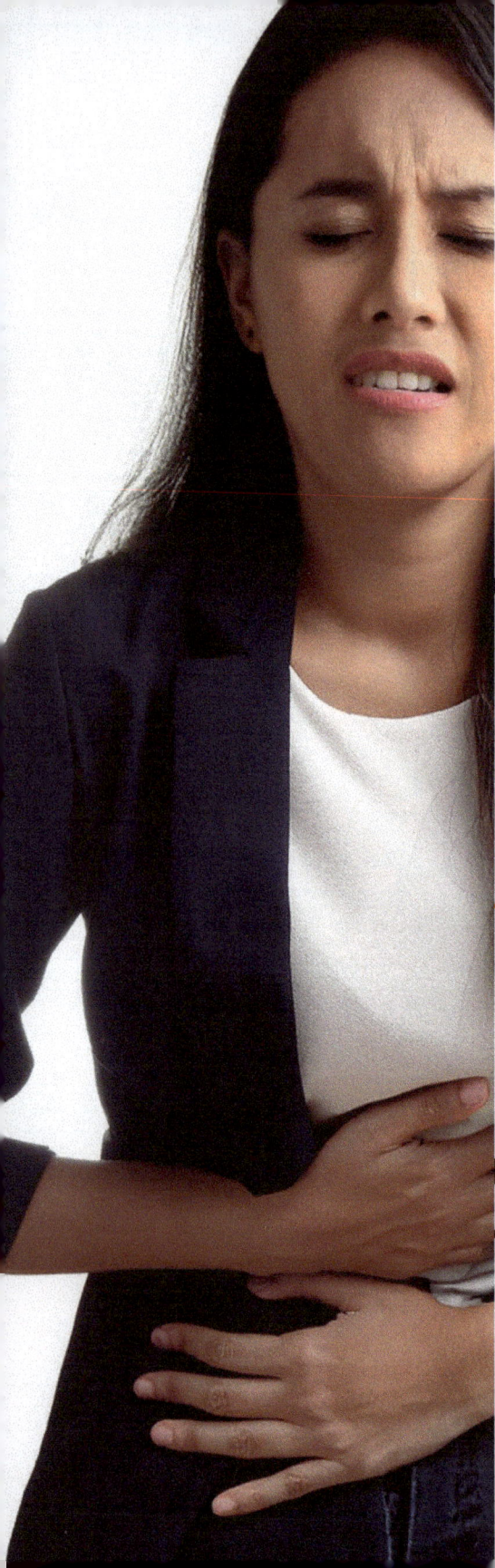

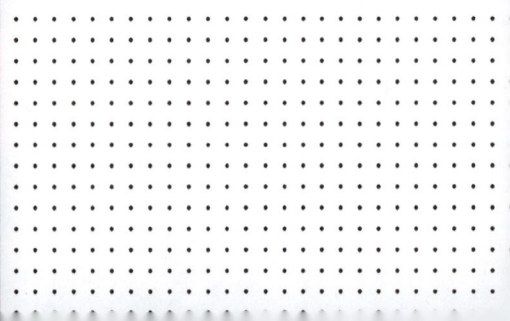

13
Vomiting

Vomiting is a protective reflex that expels contents from the stomach through the mouth. It can result from gastrointestinal, neurological, metabolic, or systemic conditions. While often benign, it can signal serious underlying diseases when associated with specific red flags or persistent symptoms. Identifying the cause and assessing the severity are critical to management.

Diagnostic sieves

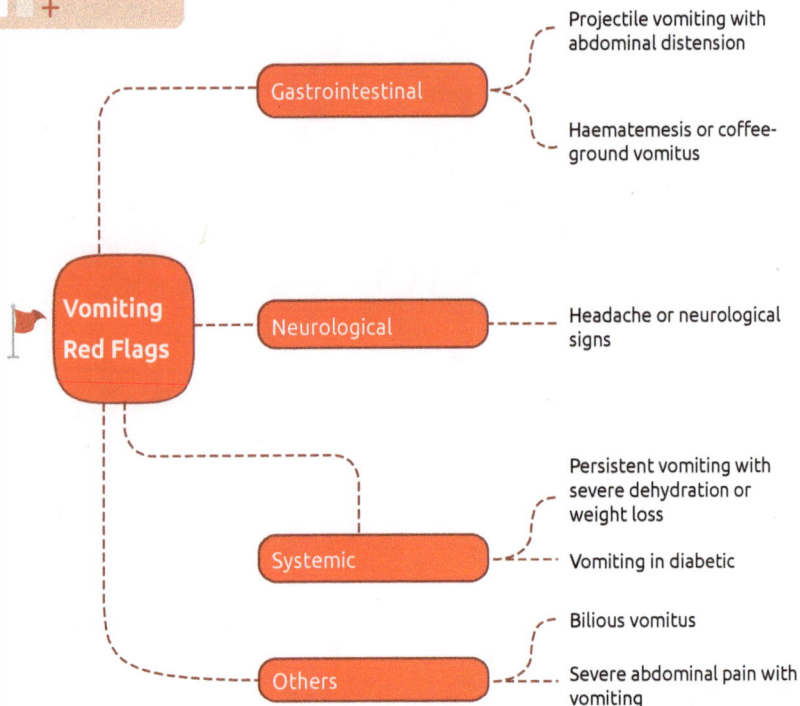

■ ▢ ▢ +

Gastrointestinal
- Projectile vomiting with abdominal distension
- Haematemesis or coffee-ground vomitus

Vomiting Red Flags

Neurological
- Headache or neurological signs

Systemic
- Persistent vomiting with severe dehydration or weight loss
- Vomiting in diabetic

Others
- Bilious vomitus
- Severe abdominal pain with vomiting

Differential diagnoses using the VITAMIN CDE framework

Category	Examples
V – Vascular	Mesenteric ischemia, ischemic bowel, raised ICP (venous sinus thrombosis).
I – Infectious	Gastroenteritis, meningitis, pyelonephritis, hepatitis.
T – Toxicological	Alcohol intoxication, drug overdose (e.g., aspirin, opioids), chemotherapy.
A – Autoimmune	Systemic lupus erythematosus (SLE), celiac disease.
M – Metabolic	Diabetic ketoacidosis (DKA), Addisonian crisis, hypercalcemia, uremia.
I – Idiopathic	Idiopathic gastroparesis, functional vomiting syndromes.
N – Neoplastic	Gastric cancer, pancreatic cancer, brain tumors (raised ICP).
C – Congenital	Pyloric stenosis, malrotation with volvulus, biliary atresia.
D – Degenerative	Chronic pancreatitis, end-stage renal disease.
E – Environmental	Motion sickness, high-altitude sickness, toxin ingestion.

History Taking

1. DURATION AND PATTERN:
How long has the vomiting been going on? How often does it occur?.

2. PRECIPITATING FACTORS:
- Triggers such as food intake, medications, or stress.

3. ASSOCIATED SYMPTOMS:
- Weight loss, abdominal pain, diarrhea, or neurological symptoms.

4. SPECIFIC FEATURES:
- Features of bowel obstruction (e.g., projectile vomiting, abdominal distension).

- Evidence of fluid depletion (e.g., pallor, hypotension, tachycardia).
- Symptoms of DKA (e.g., vomiting in a diabetic patient).
- Features of raised intracranial pressure (e.g., headache, visual changes).

5. RISK FACTORS:
- History of renal failure, pancreatitis, or gastrointestinal disorders.
- Vomit with blood or "coffee ground" material (indicates GI bleeding).
- History of pregnancy (rule out hyperemesis gravidarum).

Symptoms & Patterns

- Acute Vomiting: Common causes: Gastroenteritis, food poisoning, DKA, acute abdomen.
- Chronic or Recurrent Vomiting: Common causes: GERD, gastroparesis, chronic pancreatitis.

- Vomiting with Blood: Suggests GI bleeding (e.g., peptic ulcer, varices).
- Projectile Vomiting: Indicates obstruction (e.g., pyloric stenosis, bowel obstruction) or neurological causes (e.g., raised ICP).

Serious Diagnoses to Consider

1. ACUTE ABDOMEN:

Examples: Appendicitis, bowel obstruction, perforation.

Key Features: Severe abdominal pain, rigidity, absent bowel sounds.

Diagnostic Tools: Erect abdominal X-ray, CT abdomen.

2. DIABETIC KETOACIDOSIS (DKA):

Key Features: Nausea, vomiting, abdominal pain, hyperventilation, confusion.

Diagnostic Tools: Blood glucose, arterial blood gas (ABG), serum ketones.

3. BOWEL OBSTRUCTION:

Key Features: Projectile vomiting, absolute constipation, distended abdomen.

Diagnostic Tools: Abdominal X-ray, CT scan. Raised Intracranial Pressure (ICP):

Key Features: Vomiting with headache, visual changes, altered consciousness.

Diagnostic Tools: CT/MRI brain, fundoscopy.

4. ACUTE PANCREATITIS:

Key Features: Severe epigastric pain radiating to the back, nausea, vomiting.

Diagnostic Tools: Serum amylase/lipase, abdominal CT scan.

5. MENINGITIS:

Key Features: Fever, headache, neck stiffness, photophobia, vomiting.

Diagnostic Tools: Lumbar puncture, blood cultures.

6. HYPEREMESIS GRAVIDARUM:

Key Features: Persistent vomiting in pregnancy, weight loss, dehydration.

Diagnostic Tools: Urinalysis for ketones, serum electrolytes.

Diagnostic sieves
■ □ □ +

Serious diagnoses to consider

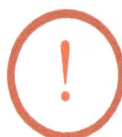

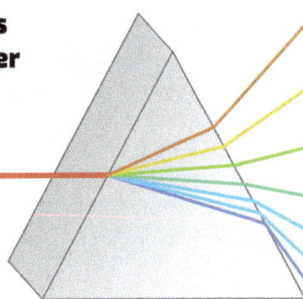

!

- Acute Abdomen
- Diabetic Ketoacidosis
- Bowel Obstruction
- Raised ICP
- Acute Pancreatitis
- Meningitis
- Hyperemesis Gravidarum

❗ SERIOUS SYMPTOMS!

- Projectile vomiting: Suggests **bowel obstruction or neurological causes** (e.g., raised ICP).
- Hematemesis or coffee-ground vomit: Indicates **upper GI bleeding.**
- Bilious vomiting: Suggests **obstruction distal to the ampulla of Vater.**
- Severe abdominal pain: Indicates acute abdomen (e.g., **perforation, pancreatitis**).
- Persistent vomiting with weight loss: Raises concerns for **malignancy** or chronic conditions like **gastroparesis.**

❗ SERIOUS SIGNS!

- Dehydration: Tachycardia, hypotension, dry mucous membranes, reduced urine output.
- Neurological deficits: Focal deficits, altered consciousness, or papilledema (**suggesting raised ICP**).
- Abdominal distension with absent bowel sounds: Indicates **bowel obstruction or paralytic ileus.**
- Jaundice with vomiting: Suggests hepatobiliary disease (e.g., **pancreatitis, cholangitis**).
- Signs of sepsis: Fever, hypotension, and tachycardia.

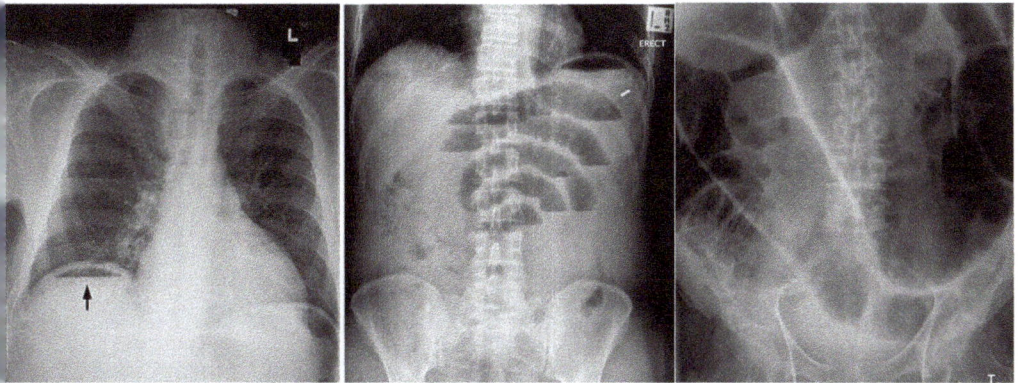

Figure 6.1: Chest XR (left) showing free air under diaphragm; (Middle) Abdominal XR showing small bowel obstruction; (right) Abdominal image showing large bowel obstruction

Are you missing something?

I. BOWEL OBSTRUCTION

Clinical features: Abdominal pain, absolute constipation, diarrhoea may be an early symptom, projectile vomiting, distended abdomen, fever, tachycardia.

Investigation:

- Erect CXR : air under diaphragm if perforation
- AXR: fluid levels
- CT abdomen

Etiology:

- Small bowel: Adhesions(55 %), strictures, hernia, IBD (10%), volvulus (3%)
- Large bowel: Strictures, diverticulitis, malignancy
- Functional (ileus):Surgery, sepsis, metabolic disturbance, drugs, immobility.

DIABETIC KETOACIDOSIS (DKA)

Metabolic acidosis secondary to an uncontrolled catabolic state due to insulin deficiency. This results in hyperketonemia and hyperglycemia. Severe fluid depletion leads to the breakdown of free fatty acids into ketones in the liver, causing acidosis and osmotic diuresis.

Clinical Features:

- Dehydration
- Abdominal pain

- Nausea and vomiting
- Hyperventilation (Kussmaul breathing)
- Confusion, malaise, and lethargy.

Mnemonic: DKA

- **D**: Diuresis (osmotic diuresis, dehydration).
- **K**: Kussmaul breathing, ketotic breath, K+ (initial hyperkalemia).
- **A**: Abdominal pain.

Important Risks

- Severe dehydration leading to circulatory collapse and shock.
- Precipitating illness such as sepsis.
- Cardiac arrest due to presenting hyperkalemia or hypokalemia after insulin therapy.
- Cerebral edema.

3. HYPEROSMOLAR HYPERGLYCEMIC STATE (HONK)

A partial insulin deficit leads to hyperglycemia. Acidosis does not occur initially due to a lack of ketogenesis. The main concern is extreme dehydration and hyperosmolarity.

Clinical Features:

- Extreme dehydration.
- Hyperglycemia without ketosis or acidosis.
- Neurological symptoms (altered mental state).

Mnemonic: HONK

- **H**: Hyperosmolarity, hypernatremia, hypercalcemia.
- **O**: No ketosis, no acidosis, no vomiting.
- **N**: Neurological symptoms, negative Gram-negative septicemia.
- **K**: Koagulation complications (DVT, DIC), K+ (hyperkalemia).

4. **ADDISONIAN CRISIS:**

Acute adrenal insufficiency leading to a deficiency in glucocorticoids and mineralocorticoids.

Tends to occur due to sudden withdrawal of steroids in patients on chronic steroid therapy. Addison's disease with crisis precipitated by illness, stress, or infections, increasing steroid demand.

Clinical Features:

- Abdominal pain and vomiting.
- Hypoglycemia.
- Shock.
- Hyperpigmentation (often chronic).

Investigations:

- Increased serum potassium and calcium.
- Decreased serum sodium.
- Assess uric acid and cortisol levels.

Top Tips

- Always consider pregnancy in women of childbearing age presenting with vomiting.
- Persistent vomiting with neurological symptoms warrants urgent imaging to exclude raised ICP.
- Projectile vomiting in infants is pyloric stenosis until proven otherwise.
- Severe dehydration can lead to circulatory collapse; assess and treat promptly.
- Bilious vomiting is an emergency; consider bowel obstruction or volvulus.
- Beware of the patient with Vomiting and a headache unless it is obviously migraine.
- Check BM in diabetics who are vomiting to rule out DKA.
- Gastroenteritis should cause increased bowel sounds. In the patient with abdominal pain and vomiting, if bowel sounds are absent or scanty, the diagnosis is likely to be an acute abdomen.

Mneumonic for causes of vomiting

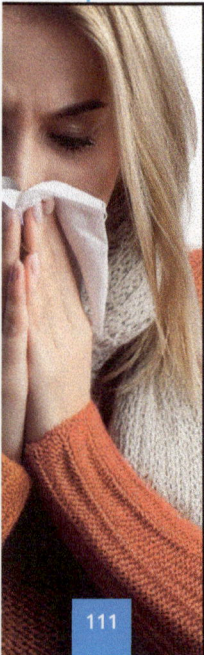

VOMITING

Vestibular/Vagal reflex (Pain)

Opiates

Migraine/Metabolic e.g. DKA

Infection

Toxicity (cytotoxic, digoxin)

Increased IOP/Ingested alcohol

Neurogenic

GI/Gestation

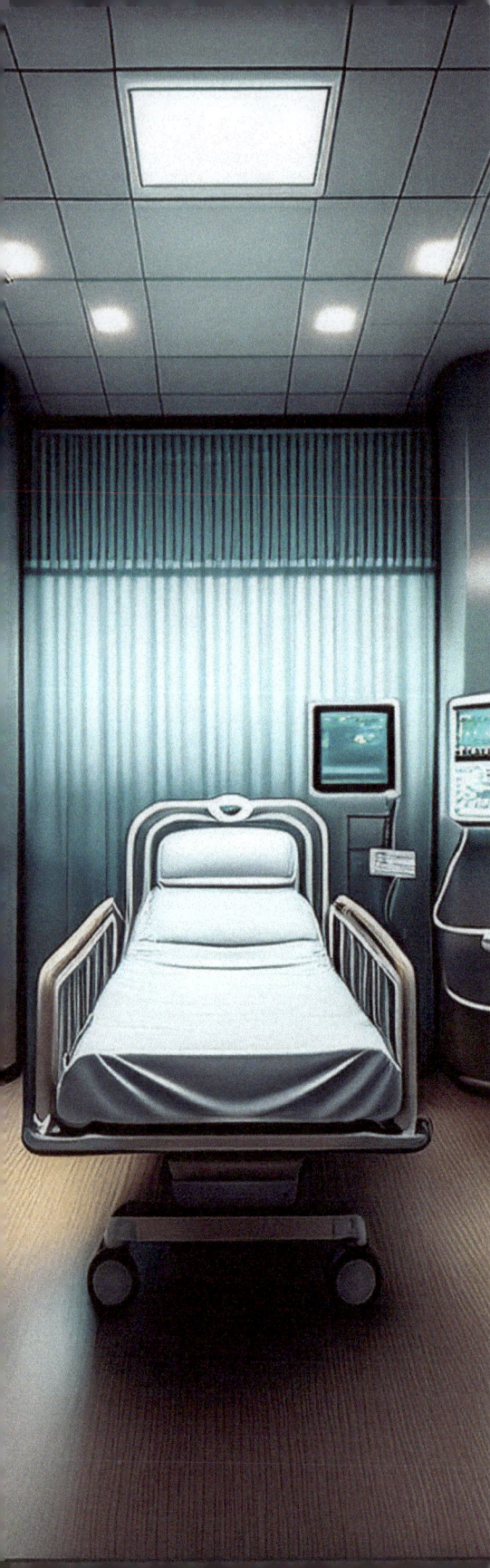

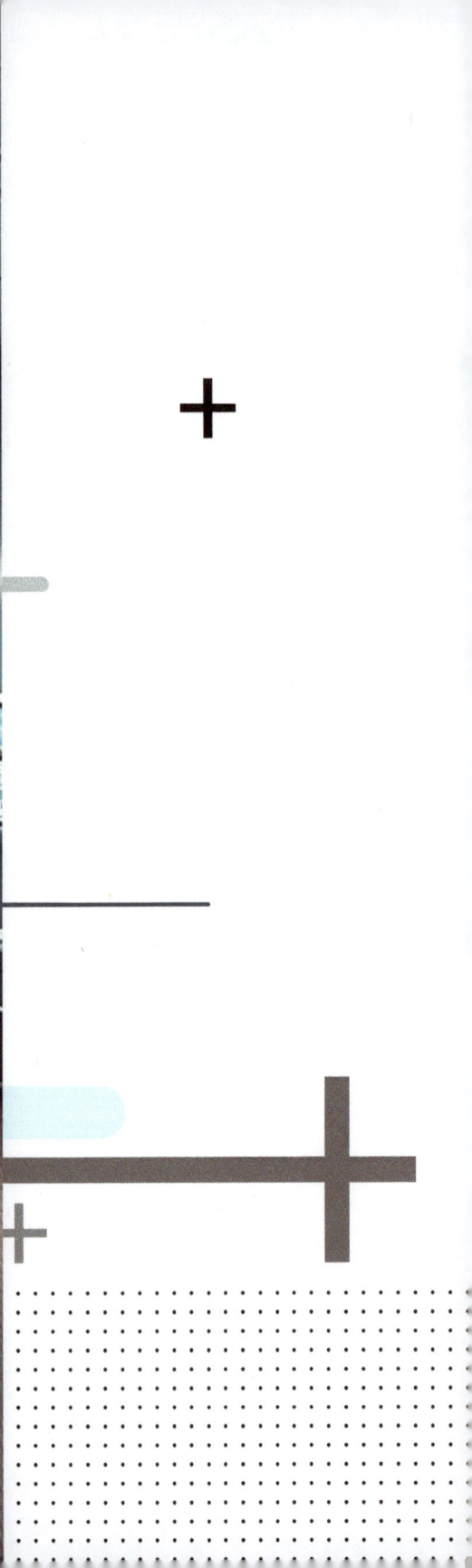

14
Haematemesis

Haematemesis, the vomiting of blood, is a medical emergency that requires rapid assessment and intervention to prevent morbidity and mortality. Causes range from benign conditions such as Mallory-Weiss tears to life-threatening oesophageal varices or malignancies. Key clues include the nature of the bleeding (bright red vs. coffee-ground vomitus), associated symptoms, and risk factors such as NSAID use, alcohol consumption, or liver disease. A structured approach to history, examination, and the use of risk stratification scores, such as the Glasgow-Blatchford or Rockall score, ensures accurate diagnosis and timely management.

Diagnostic sieves

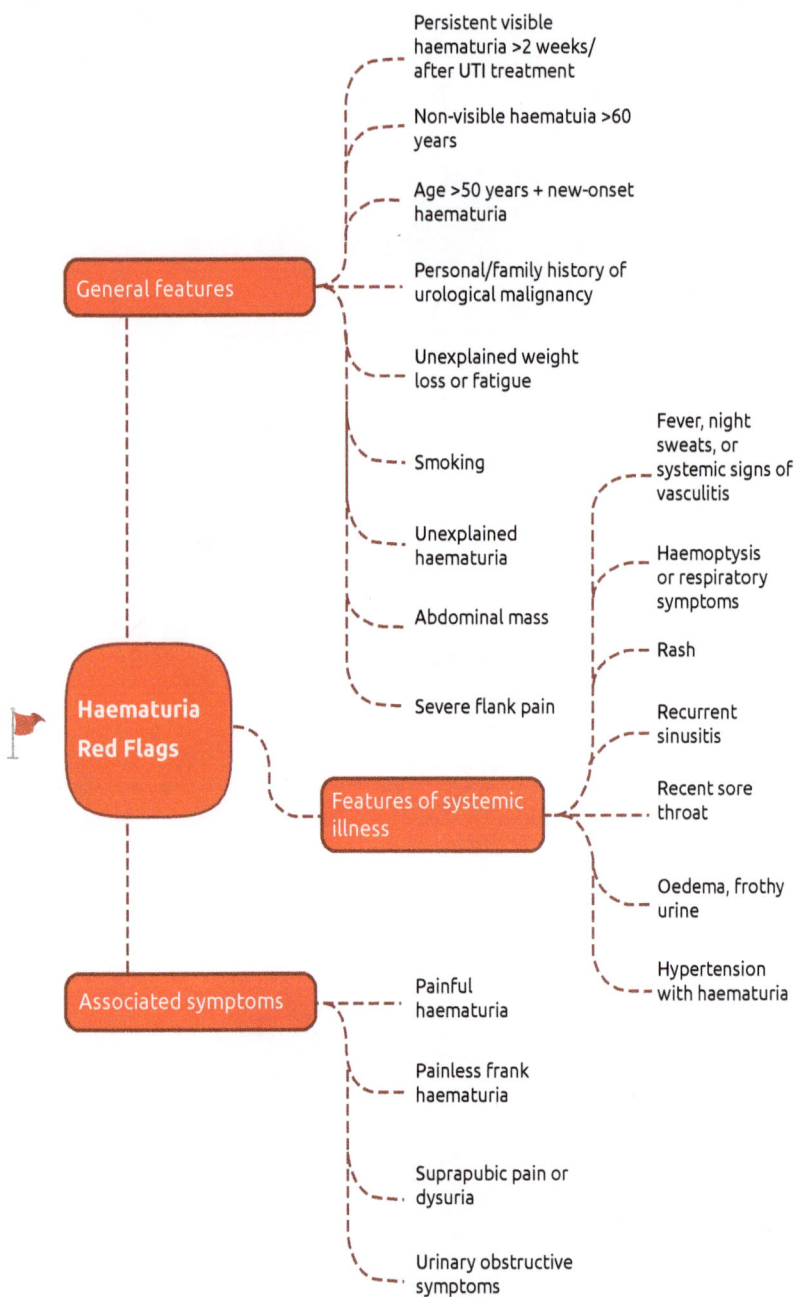

■ □ □ +

Haematuria Red Flags

General features

- Persistent visible haematuria >2 weeks/ after UTI treatment
- Non-visible haematuia >60 years
- Age >50 years + new-onset haematuria
- Personal/family history of urological malignancy
- Unexplained weight loss or fatigue
- Smoking
- Unexplained haematuria
- Abdominal mass
- Severe flank pain

Features of systemic illness

- Fever, night sweats, or systemic signs of vasculitis
- Haemoptysis or respiratory symptoms
- Rash
- Recurrent sinusitis
- Recent sore throat
- Oedema, frothy urine
- Hypertension with haematuria

Associated symptoms

- Painful haematuria
- Painless frank haematuria
- Suprapubic pain or dysuria
- Urinary obstructive symptoms

History Taking - Important points

1. DURATION OF SYMPTOMS
- Acute bleeding often points to peptic ulcers, Mallory-Weiss tears, or oesophageal varices.
- Chronic or intermittent episodes might indicate more insidious causes like malignancy, gastric or oesophageal cancer, or chronic gastritis.

2. ALCOHOL CONSUMPTION
- Chronic alcohol use increases the risk of liver disease and portal hypertension, which can lead to oesophageal varices and significant bleeding. It also raises the likelihood of gastritis or peptic ulcers.

3. MEDICATIONS (NSAIDS, ANTICOAGU-LANTS)
- NSAID use can predispose to peptic ulcers and erosive gastritis, while anticoagulants increase the risk of spontaneous bleeding, including from varices or ulcers.

4. HISTORY OF LIVER DISEASE OR PORTAL HYPERTENSION
- Liver disease, particularly cirrhosis, can lead to portal hypertension and oesophageal varices, which are major causes of upper gastrointestinal bleeding. Signs of ascites, jaundice, or encephalopathy may further suggest portal hypertension.

5. EPIGASTRIC PAIN OR HEARTBURN
- Epigastric pain, especially when associated with haematemesis, is characteristic of peptic ulcers or gastritis. Heartburn may indicate acid reflux or erosive oesophagitis, which can lead to haemorrhagic complications.

6. HISTORY OF WEIGHT LOSS OR DYS-PHAGIA
- Unexplained weight loss and dysphagia are red flags for malignancy, particularly oesophageal or gastric cancer. These symptoms, when associated with haematemesis, raise concern for advanced malignancy.

7. RECENT VOMITING
- Forceful vomiting before haematemesis suggests a Mallory-Weiss tear, commonly seen after episodes of retching or vomiting. This is typically a benign but painful cause of bleeding.

8. COAGULATION DISORDERS (E.G., ANTICOAGULANT THERAPY)
- Coagulopathy increases the risk of gastrointestinal bleeding. A history of anticoagulant use or clotting disorders should raise suspicion for spontaneous bleeding from peptic ulcers, oesophageal varices, or other lesions.

9. FAMILY HISTORY OF CANCER OR CO-AGULATION DISORDERS
- A family history of gastrointestinal cancer or bleeding disorders increases the suspicion for inherited risks, such as oesophageal or gastric cancer, or bleeding conditions like hereditary coagulopathies

Are you missing something?

- **Oesophageal varices** due to their high mortality.
- **Perforated peptic ulcers** leading to peritonitis.
- **Malignancies** causing insidious upper GI bleeding.

Top tips

CLINICAL PATTERNS TO NOTE
- Bright red blood often indicates active variceal or arterial bleeding.
- Coffee-ground vomitus suggests slower

Diagnostic sieves

Serious diagnoses to consider

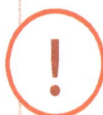

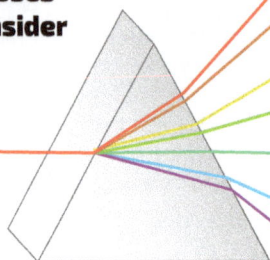

Gastrointestinal Malignancies (Gastric or Oesophageal Cancer)

Oesophageal Varices

Peptic Ulcer Disease with active bleeding

Mallory-Weiss Tear

Boerhaave's Syndrome (Ruptured Oesophagus)

Erosive Oesophagitis or Gastritis

Coagulopathies or Bleeding Disorders

SERIOUS SYMPTOMS!

- Painless haematemesis: Suggests **oesophageal varices or malignancy.**
- Epigastric pain with haematemesis: Likely **peptic ulcer disease or erosive gastritis.**
- Vomiting followed by blood: **Mallory-Weiss tear.**
- Jaundice and ascites with haematemesis: Indicative of **portal hypertension and variceal bleeding.**
- Persistent weight loss and dysphagia: Suggests **upper GI malignancy.**
- Coffee-ground vomitus: Suggests slower **upper GI bleeding.**

SERIOUS SIGNS!

- Flank tenderness or palpable mass: May indicate **malignancy or large ulcers.**
- Signs of systemic illness: Fever, rash, or arthritis (consider **vasculitis or infection**).
- Hypotension or tachycardia: Suggests significant b**lood loss.**
- Jaundice and spider naevi: Indicate **chronic liver disease and possible varices.**
- Significant proteinuria or haematuria: Raises suspicion of **systemic vasculitis.**

Differential diagnosis of haematemesis

Category	Examples
V – Vascular	Oesophageal varices, Mallory-Weiss tear.
I – Infectious	*H. pylori*-related ulcers, oesophagitis.
T – Trauma	Boerhaave's syndrome, prolonged retching.
A – Autoimmune	Vasculitis (e.g., Behçet's disease).
M – Metabolic	Portal hypertension, alcohol-related gastritis.
I – Iatrogenic	NSAID or anticoagulant-related bleeding.
N – Neoplastic	Gastric or oesophageal malignancy.
D – Degenerative	Peptic ulcer disease, erosive gastritis.
C – Congenital	Rare structural lesions like Dieulafoy's lesion.

Admission risk marker	Score value
Blood urea (mmol/L)	
6.5–8	2
8–10	3
10–25	4
>25	6
Hb (g/L) for men	
120–130	1
100–120	3
<100	6
Hb (g/L) for women	
100–120	1
<100	6
Systolic blood pressure (mmHg)	
100–109	1
90–99	2
<90	3
Pulse ≥100/minute	1
History/co-morbidities	
Presentation with melaena	1
Presentation with syncope	2
Hepatic disease*	2
Cardiac failure†	2

*Known history of or clinical/laboratory evidence of chronic or acute liver disease
†Known history of or clinical/echocardiographic evidence of cardiac failure

Figure 17.1
researchgate.net/figure/Glasgow-Blatchford-score-GBS_tbl2_51601749

or less acute bleeding.
- Melena often accompanies significant haematemesis.

APPROACH TO DIAGNOSIS

- Use risk stratification scores like the Glasgow-Blatchford or Rockall score.
- Perform urgent OGD for suspected variceal or arterial bleeding.
- Distinguish haematemesis from epistaxis or haemoptysis using history and examination.

Glasgow Blatchford Score

The Glasgow Blatchford Score (GBS; left)) assesses the severity of upper gastrointestinal bleeding at presentation and helps identify patients who may be safely managed as outpatients without the need for urgent endoscopy: 0: Low risk (may be safely managed as outpatient), 1-4: Moderate risk, ≥5: High risk (requires urgent endoscopy).

The Rockall Score

The Rockall score (next page) helps predict the risk of rebleeding and mortality, guiding clinical decisions on management, including whether to admit the patient or manage them conservatively.

In summary:
- Predicts the risk of rebleeding and mortality.
- Helps guide clinical decisions on admission and conservative vs. interventional management.

	0	1	2	3
Age	<60	60-79	>80	
BP & HR	BP > 100 HR < 100	BP > 100 HR > 100	BP < 100	
Co-morbidites	None	-	CCF / IHD major co-morbity	AKI, Liver failure, metastatic Ca
Diagonsis	Mallory-Weiss / no pathology	All other	Malignancy	
Bleeding on endoscopy?	None of dark spots only	-	Blood clot, Spurting vessel	

Figure 17.2: The Rockall score
app.pulsenotes.com/medicine/gastroenterology/notes/upper-gi-bleeding

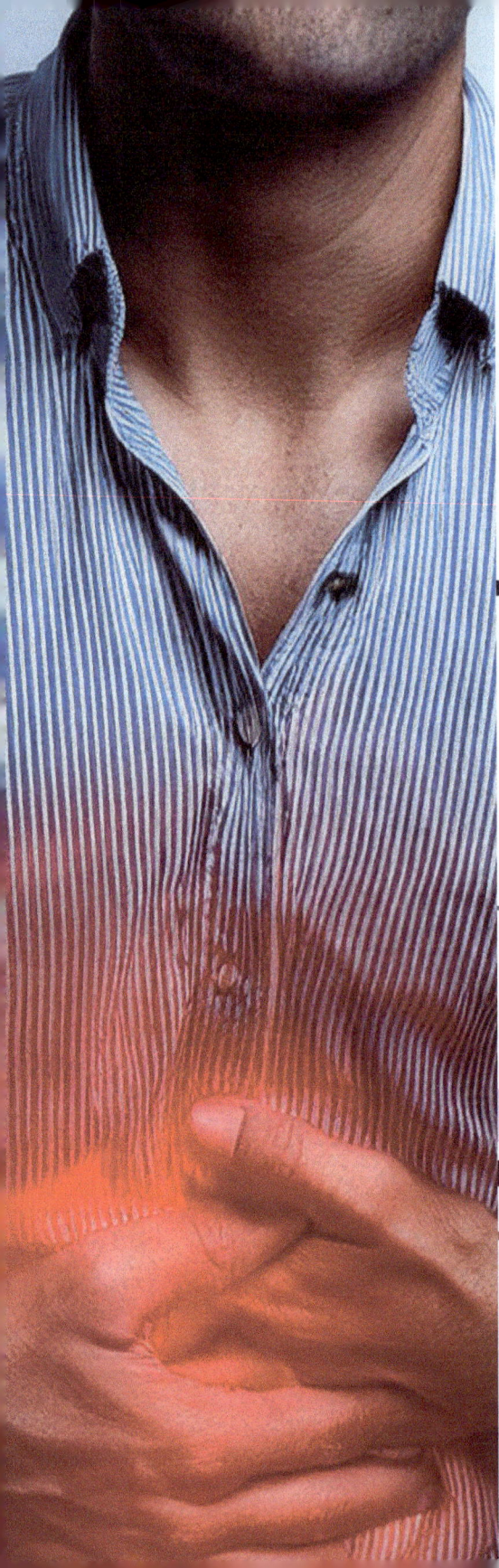

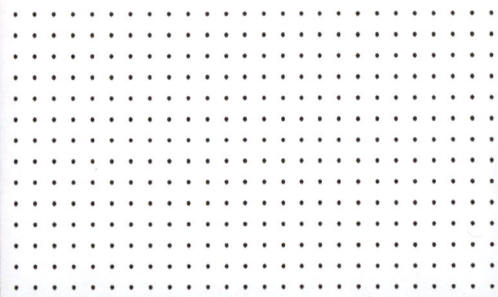

15

Rectal Bleeding

Rectal bleeding is a common clinical presentation, defined as the passage of blood through the rectum, which can range from minor spotting to life-threatening hemorrhage. The causes span benign conditions like hemorrhoids to serious, life-threatening diseases such as colorectal cancer or ischemic colitis. Identifying the source of bleeding is crucial, as the management varies significantly depending on the underlying etiology. Recognizing red flags, systemic symptoms, and associated gastrointestinal or systemic conditions is key to accurate diagnosis and timely intervention

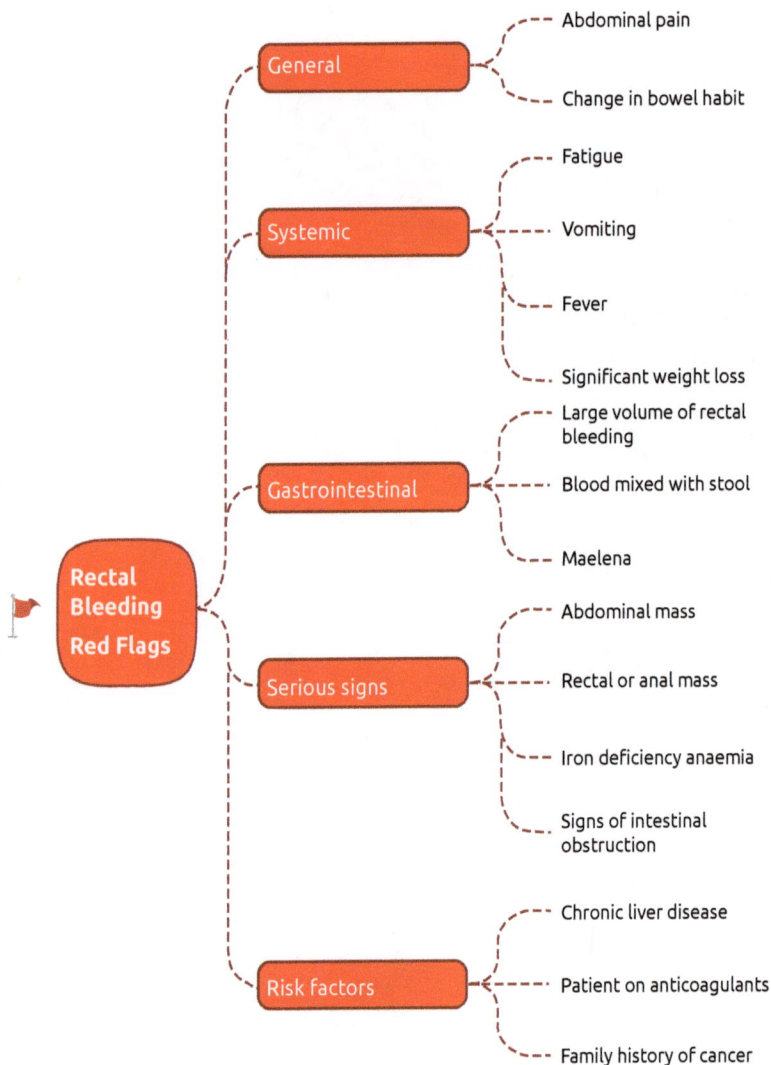

Rectal Bleeding Red Flags

- **General**
  - Abdominal pain
  - Change in bowel habit
- **Systemic**
  - Fatigue
  - Vomiting
  - Fever
  - Significant weight loss
- **Gastrointestinal**
  - Large volume of rectal bleeding
  - Blood mixed with stool
  - Maelena
- **Serious signs**
  - Abdominal mass
  - Rectal or anal mass
  - Iron deficiency anaemia
  - Signs of intestinal obstruction
- **Risk factors**
  - Chronic liver disease
  - Patient on anticoagulants
  - Family history of cancer

History Taking - Important points

Is it acute or chronic?

- This distinguishes sudden-onset conditions, which are often associated with ischaemia, diverticular disease, or infectious colitis, from long-standing issues like haemorrhoids, colorectal cancer, or IBD.

Is the bleeding painful?

- Painful bleeding often suggests haemorrhoids, anal fissures, or anal canal cancer, whereas painless bleeding is more typical of conditions like polyps, Meckel's diverticulum, or colorectal malignancies.

Is the bleeding associated with tenesmus?

- The presence of tenesmus indicates irritation or inflammation in the rectal or colonic lining and is suggestive of conditions like rectal cancer, ulcerative colitis, or post-radiation proctitis.

What is the nature of the blood in relation to stools?

- Blood splashing or dripping after defecation is consistent with haemorrhoids, while blood streaked on stool suggests anal or rectal cancer. Mixed blood and stool often point to colonic lesions.

What is the colour of the blood?

- Bright red blood indicates a distal source like the rectum or anal canal, while maroon stools suggest bleeding from the small intestine. Black stools, or melena, signify an upper GI bleed, and streaked brown stools with blood are indicative of rectosigmoid involvement.

Is there weight loss, anorexia, or vomiting?

- These systemic symptoms strongly suggest malignancy, particularly colorectal cancer, and should always raise concern for serious pathology requiring further investigation.

Is the patient on anticoagulants?
Is there any family history of cancer?
Is there a history of chronic liver disease?

- Chronic liver disease raises the possibility of variceal bleeding.

Are you missing something?

- **Colorectal cancer:** Be vigilant for rectal bleeding, weight loss, abdominal pain, and changes in bowel habits, especially in patients over 50.
- **Ischaemic colitis or mesenteric ischaemia:** Look for severe rectal bleeding, abdominal pain, and a history of vascular risk factors.
- **Diverticular disease with bleeding:** Particularly in elderly patients, diverticulosis can present with acute, severe bleeding.

Top tips

CLINICAL PATTERNS TO NOTE

- Fresh bright red blood on the toilet paper usually comes from perianal sources (e.g., haemorrhoids or fissures).
- Blood mixed with stool usually indicates a higher GI tract source (e.g., colonic or rectal cancer).
- Weight loss and anorexia with rectal bleeding raises concern for malignancy.
- Chronic, recurrent rectal bleeding should prompt investigation for IBD, polyps, or colorectal cancer, especially if the patient is over 50 years old.

APPROACH TO DIAGNOSIS

First, **rule out life-threatening conditions** such as colorectal cancer, ischaemic colitis, or major bleeding.

Serious diagnoses to consider

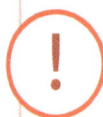

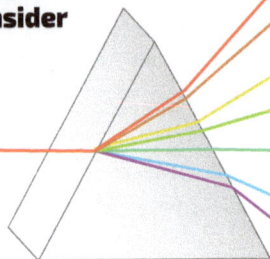

(!)

Colorectal Carcinoma

Rectal Carcinoma

Cholangiocarcinoma

Inflammatory Bowel Disease (IBD)

Ischaemic Colitis

Infectious Colitis (e.g. C. difficile, bacterial infections)

Mesenteric Ischaemia

! SERIOUS SYMPTOMS!

- Rectal bleeding in elderly patients — suggestive of **colorectal carcinoma**.
- Large volume of blood mixed with stool — indicative of **inflammatory bowel disease (IBD), colorectal cancer, or severe diverticular disease**.
- Painless rectal bleeding with significant weight loss, anorexia, or fatigue — raises concern for **malignancy, such as colorectal carcinoma**.
- Change in bowel habits — suggestive of **colorectal cancer, diverticular disease, or IBD**.
- Chronic liver disease — increases the risk of variceal bleeding, often presenting as significant rectal bleeding.
- Use of anticoagulants — heightens the risk of significant bleeding, particularly in conditions such as diverticular disease or angiodysplasia.

! SERIOUS SIGNS!

- Signs of intestinal obstruction, including abdominal distension, vomiting, and constipation — suggestive of colorectal cancer, intussusception, or mesenteric thrombosis.
- Iron deficiency anaemia — indicative of chronic blood loss from malignancies such as colorectal or gastric carcinoma.
- Black tarry stools or maroon-coloured stools — suggestive of upper gastrointestinal bleeding or small bowel bleeding, respectively.
- Abdominal masses or palpable rectal masses — strongly indicative of colorectal or rectal cancer.
- Reduced urine output and other signs of shock (e.g., tachycardia, hypotension) — suggest severe blood loss from mesenteric ischaemia or massive gastrointestinal bleeding.

Initial diagnostic approach may include:

- Rectal examination: To assess for haemorrhoids, fissures, or palpable masses.

- Endoscopy (colonoscopy or sigmoidoscopy): To identify and biopsy suspicious lesions.

Differential diagnoses of rectal bleeding

Category	Differential Diagnoses
V - Vascular	Ischemic colitis, Mesenteric ischemia (acute or chronic), Angiodysplasia, Diverticular disease
I - Infectious	Gastroenteritis (bacterial/viral), Clostridium difficile infection, HIV-related infections
T - Trauma	Post-radiation proctitis, Trauma-induced hemorrhage (e.g., anal trauma)
A - Autoimmune	Inflammatory bowel disease (Crohn's disease, ulcerative colitis)
M - Metabolic	Anticoagulant therapy (e.g., warfarin, DOACs)
I - Idiopathic	Angiodysplasia
N - Neoplastic	Colorectal cancer, Rectal cancer, Other gastrointestinal malignancies (e.g., gastric carcinoma)
D - Degenerative	Diverticular disease (with complications)
C - Congenital	Meckel's diverticulum

Type of Bleeding	Percentage of Cases
Colonic Bleeding	
Diverticular Disease	40%
Ischaemic Colitis	10-20%
Colorectal Cancer	10-20%
Inflammatory Bowel Disease (IBD)	10%
Angiodysplasia	5-10%
Haemorrhoids	10-15%
Post-Polypectomy Bleeding	5-10%
Small Bowel Bleeding	
Angiodysplasia	50%
Neoplasms	10-20%
Small Bowel Ulcers	10-20%
Crohn's Disease	10-20%
Meckel's Diverticulum	5-10%

The table above categorizes rectal bleeding presentations by source of bleeding;
https://academic.oup.com/ibdjournal/article/27/11/1773/6058971
https://academic.oup.com/gastro/article/2/4/300/2910197

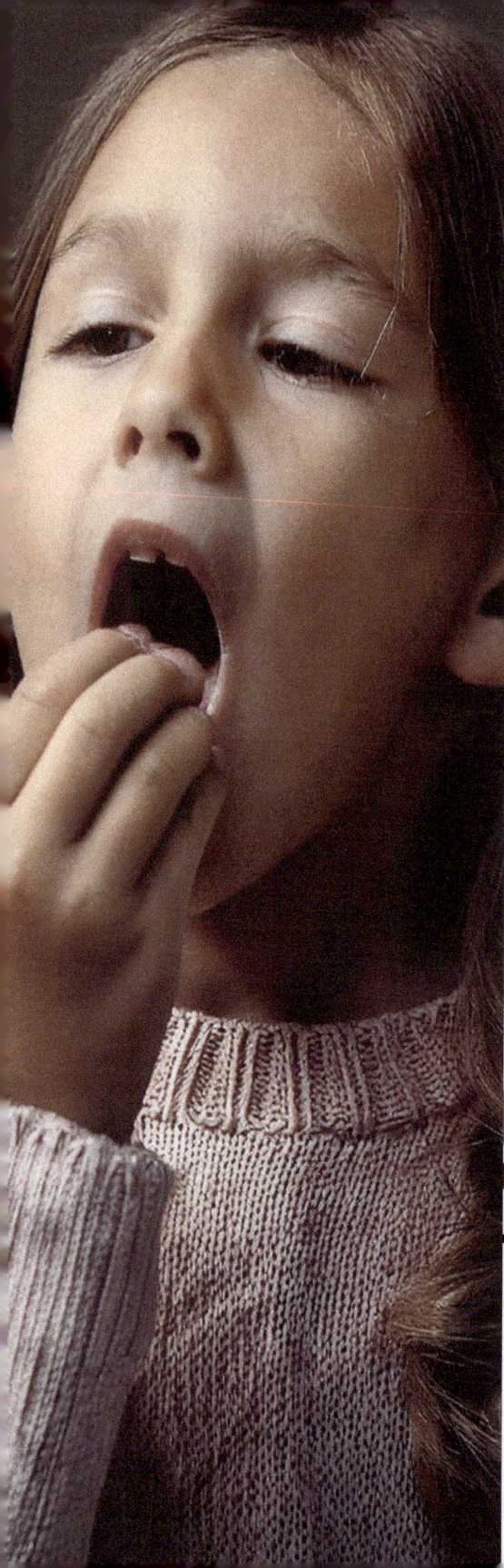

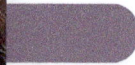

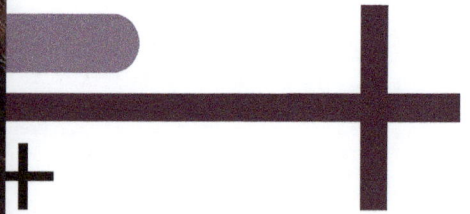

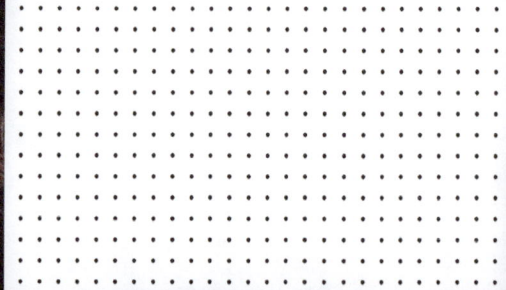

16

Dysphagia

Dysphagia or difficulty swallowing, is a symptom that can arise from a wide range of conditions, spanning benign functional disorders to serious, life-threatening illnesses. It may affect the swallowing of solids, liquids, or both, and its presentation offers important clues to its underlying cause. Proper identification and investigation are essential, especially in cases with progressive symptoms, associated weight loss, or red flag features, as these may indicate malignancy or neurological disorders requiring urgent intervention.

Dysphagia Red Flags

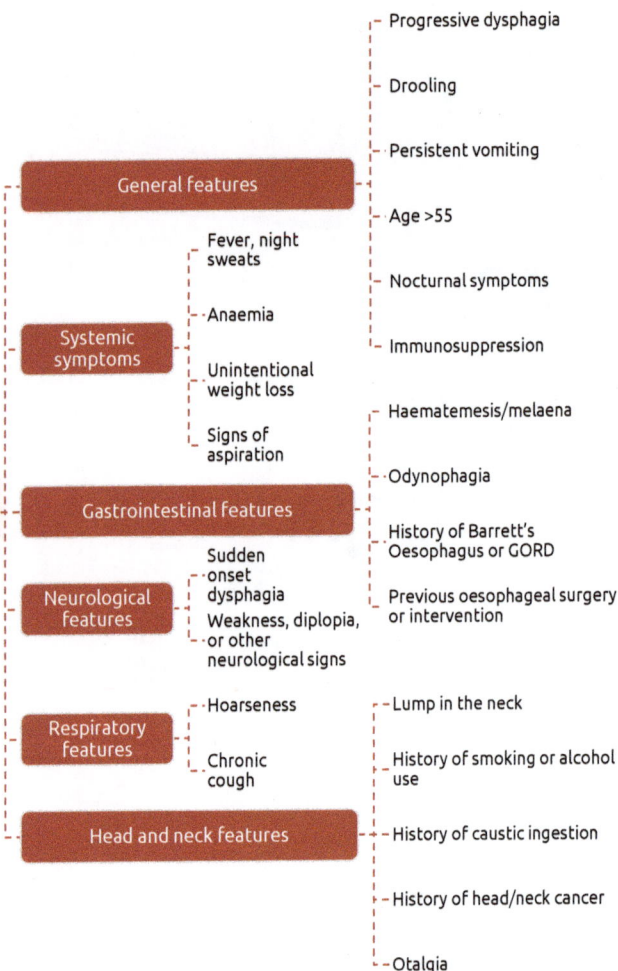

General features
- Progressive dysphagia
- Drooling
- Persistent vomiting
- Age >55
- Nocturnal symptoms
- Immunosuppression

Systemic symptoms
- Fever, night sweats
- Anaemia
- Unintentional weight loss
- Signs of aspiration

Gastrointestinal features
- Haematemesis/melaena
- Odynophagia
- History of Barrett's Oesophagus or GORD
- Previous oesophageal surgery or intervention

Neurological features
- Sudden onset dysphagia
- Weakness, diplopia, or other neurological signs

Respiratory features
- Hoarseness
- Chronic cough

Head and neck features
- Lump in the neck
- History of smoking or alcohol use
- History of caustic ingestion
- History of head/neck cancer
- Otalgia

History Taking - Important points

I. DURATION OF SYMPTOMS

- Acute onset: Likely a neurological cause (e.g., stroke, recent trauma).
- Chronic progression: Consider malignancy (e.g., oesophageal or gastric cancer), motility disorders (e.g., achalasia, scleroderma).
- Intermittent: Suggests mechanical obstruction (e.g., oesophageal rings or webs).

2. NATURE OF DIFFICULTY SWALLOWING

- Solids only: Suggests mechanical obstruction, such as oesophageal strictures, tumours, or foreign bodies.
- Liquids and solids: Indicates motility disorder, such as achalasia, scleroderma, or a neurological issue (e.g., stroke).
- Both solid and liquid difficulty: May indicate advanced disease or a neurological cause like a stroke or neurodegenerative condition (e.g., Parkinson's disease).

3. ASSOCIATED SYMPTOMS

- Heartburn or epigastric pain: Suggests gastroesophageal reflux disease (GORD), peptic ulcers, or oesophageal stricture.
- Weight loss: Raises suspicion for malignancy (e.g., oesophageal or gastric cancer).
- Neurological symptoms (e.g., weakness, dysphasia, or balance issues): Indicates a neurological cause such as a CVA or myasthenia gravis.
- Chest pain: Consider oesophageal spasm or motility disorder.
- Coughing or choking with swallowing: Suggests oropharyngeal dysphagia, commonly from neurological issues like a stroke, Parkinson's, or myasthenia gravis.

4. PRECIPITATING OR EXACERBATING FACTORS

- Cold or hot foods: Suggests a motor disorder, such as achalasia or other oesophageal motility disorders.
- Medications: Consider anticholinergics, sedatives, iron supplements, or chemotherapy agents, which can contribute to swallowing difficulty.
- Recent weight loss: Raises concern for malignancy or severe oesophageal disease.

5. RED FLAGS TO ELICIT

- New-onset dysphagia in patients >40 years: Always suspect malignancy, particularly oesophageal or gastric cancer.
- Persistent symptoms with weight loss: Likely indicates malignancy.
- Blood in vomit or stools: May point to oesophageal varices, malignancy, or gastrointestinal bleeding.
- Smoking or heavy alcohol use: Increases the risk for oesophageal or gastric cancer.

Are you missing something?

I. OESOPHAGEAL CARCINOMA

Suspect in elderly patients with progressive dysphagia and weight loss, especially those over 40 with new-onset symptoms.

2. NEUROLOGICAL CAUSES

Conditions like bulbar palsy or motor neurone disease (MND) can cause dysphagia, especially with difficulty initiating swallowing, nasal regurgitation, and aspiration following coughing.

3. EXTRINSIC COMPRESSION

Consider mediastinal tumours or thyroid goitre if there is a history of progressive dysphagia despite normal endoscopy.

4. ACHALASIA

This should be considered in patients with difficulty swallowing both solids and liquids, and who may experience regurgitation of undigested food.

Diagnostic sieves

Serious diagnoses to consider

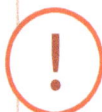

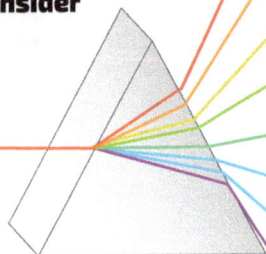

Neurological Causes: Stroke, Parkinson's Disease, Multiple Sclerosis, Myasthenia Gravis, Motor Neuron Disease

Malignancies: Esophageal or Gastric Cancer

Benign Obstruction: Strictures (e.g., from reflux or radiotherapy), Oesophageal Web, Schatzki's Ring

External Compression: Mediastinal masses, Aortic Aneurysm

Motility Disorders: Achalasia, Diffuse Oesophageal Spasm, Scleroderma

Infectious Oesophagitis e.g., Candida, CMV, HSV in immunocompromised patients

Eosinophilic Oesophagitis

Foreign Body Ingestion

SERIOUS SYMPTOMS!

- Progressive Dysphagia- red flag for malignancy or stricture.
- Odynophagia: Often seen in infections, malignancy, or severe inflammation.
- Weight Loss: Suggestive of malignancy, chronic disease, or severe obstruction
- Regurgitation of Undigested Food: Seen in achalasia or esophageal diverticula.
- Hoarseness or Voice Changes: May indicate recurrent laryngeal nerve involvement from a tumor.
- Nocturnal Cough or Aspiration: Suggestive of motility disorders like achalasia or significant obstruction.
- Chest Pain: May occur in esophageal spasm or malignancy.

SERIOUS SIGNS!

- Signs of Malignancy: Cachexia, lymphadenopathy, palpable abdominal mass.
- Respiratory Signs: Signs of aspiration pneumonia (e.g., fever, tachypnea, hypoxia) in severe dysphagia or neurological disorders.
- Oral or Pharyngeal Findings: Ulcers, masses, or candidiasis suggesting infective or neoplastic causes.
- Neurological Signs: Cranial nerve deficits, limb weakness, or coordination problems indicating underlying neurological disorders.
- Visible or Palpable Mass: Neck or mediastinal mass causing obstruction.
- Signs of Chronic Reflux: Dental erosion, hoarseness, or pharyngitis indicating GERD complications (e.g., Barrett's esophagus).

Differential diagnoses of dysphagia

Category	Conditions
V - Vascular	Oesophageal varices, Aortic aneurysm
I - Infectious and Inflammatory	Pharyngitis, Candida oesophagitis, Herpes simplex virus (HSV) oesophagitis, Tuberculosis, Eosinophilic oesophagitis
T - Trauma/Toxic	Medication-induced dysphagia, Oesophageal perforation, Radiation-induced oesophagitis
A - Autoimmune	Scleroderma, Systemic lupus erythematosus (SLE) with oesophageal involvement
M - Metabolic	Hypothyroidism, Diabetes (autonomic neuropathy), Hypercalcaemia
I - Idiopathic	Achalasia, Functional dysphagia
N - Neoplastic	Oesophageal carcinoma, Gastric carcinoma, Mediastinal tumors (e.g., lung cancer, lymphoma)
D - Degenerative	Motor neurone disease (MND), Parkinson's disease, Bulbar palsy
C - Congenital/Structural	Benign oesophageal stricture, Oesophageal webs/rings, Zenker's diverticulum

Some Helpful Findings in Dysphagia

Finding	Possible Cause
Tremor, ataxia, balance disturbance	Parkinson disease
Focal easy fatigability, particularly of facial muscles	Myasthenia gravis
Muscle fasciculation, wasting, weakness	Motor neuron disease, myopathy
Rapidly progressive, constant dysphagia, no neurologic findings	Esophageal obstruction, probably cancer
Food impaction	Eosinophilic esophagitis
Gastrointestinal reflux symptoms	Peptic stricture
Intermittent dysphagia	Lower esophageal ring or diffuse esophageal spasm
Slow progression (months to years) of dysphagia to solids and then to liquids, sometimes with nocturnal regurgitation	Achalasia
Neck mass, thyromegaly	Extrinsic compression
Dusky, erythematous rash, muscle tenderness	Dermatomyositis
Raynaud phenomenon, arthralgias, skin tightening/contractures of fingers	Systemic sclerosis
Cough, dyspnea, lung congestions	Pulmonary aspiration

Figure 22.1: From the MSD Manual Professional Version (Known as the Merck Manual in the US and Canada and the MSD Manual in the rest of the world), edited by Robert Porter. Copyright (year at bottom of web page, 2020) by Merck Sharp & Dohme Corp., a subsidiary of Merck & Co., Inc., Kenilworth, NJ.
Available at http://www.msdmanuals.com/professional. Accessed (06/03/20)

5. OESOPHAGEAL STRICTURES

Look for a history of gastro-oesophageal reflux disease (GORD) or peptic ulcer disease, which can lead to benign strictures.

Top tips

CLINICAL PATTERNS TO NOTE

- Young, anxious patients with dysphagia should be assessed for globus hystericus, a benign condition often exacerbated by stress or anxiety.
- Difficulty swallowing solids often points to mechanical obstruction, such as benign strictures or oesophageal carcinoma.
- Difficulty swallowing liquids suggests a neurological disorder, such as bulbar palsy or MND, particularly if associated with symptoms like drooling or aspiration.
- Progressive dysphagia with associated weight loss in an older adult is highly suggestive of oesophageal cancer until proven otherwise.

APPROACH TO DIAGNOSIS

- Endoscopy should be the first-line diagnostic tool to rule out structural causes such as malignancy or benign strictures.
- If endoscopy is negative, consider neurological causes or extrinsic compression, and obtain biopsies to rule out eosinophilic oesophagitis.
- Dysphagia with drooling or difficulty initiating swallowing should prompt evaluation for oropharyngeal dysphagia, possibly related to neurological disorders.
- For new-onset dysphagia in a patient with a stable long-standing neurological disorder, consider an alternate aetiology or complication.
- Patients with oesophageal dysphagia often report a sensation of food getting "stuck" after swallowing, typically in the chest or lower throat, suggesting a motility or obstructive issue.

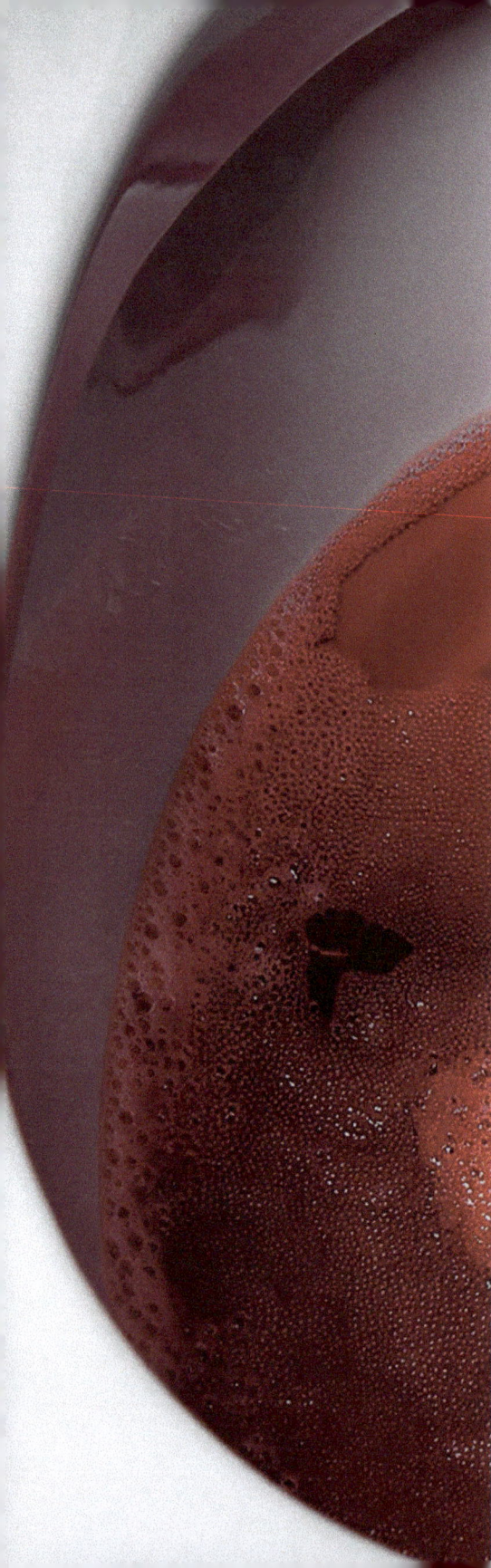

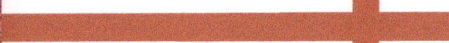

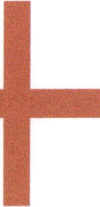

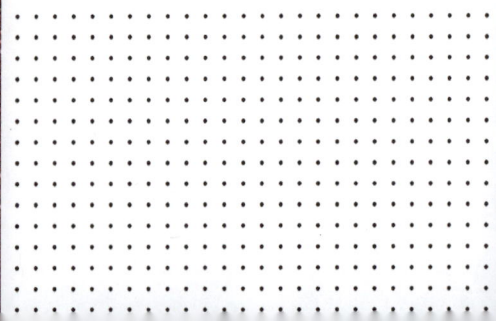

17

Haematuria

Haematuria, the presence of blood in urine, is a significant clinical symptom that can signal a range of underlying conditions, from benign causes such as a UTI to life-threatening malignancies or renal vasculitis. It can manifest as macroscopic (visible) or microscopic (non-visible) haematuria. Proper evaluation, incorporating a thorough history, examination, and targeted investigations, is essential to identify red flags, differentiate between glomerular and non-glomerular sources, and guide timely management to prevent complications or missed diagnoses.

Diagnostic sieves

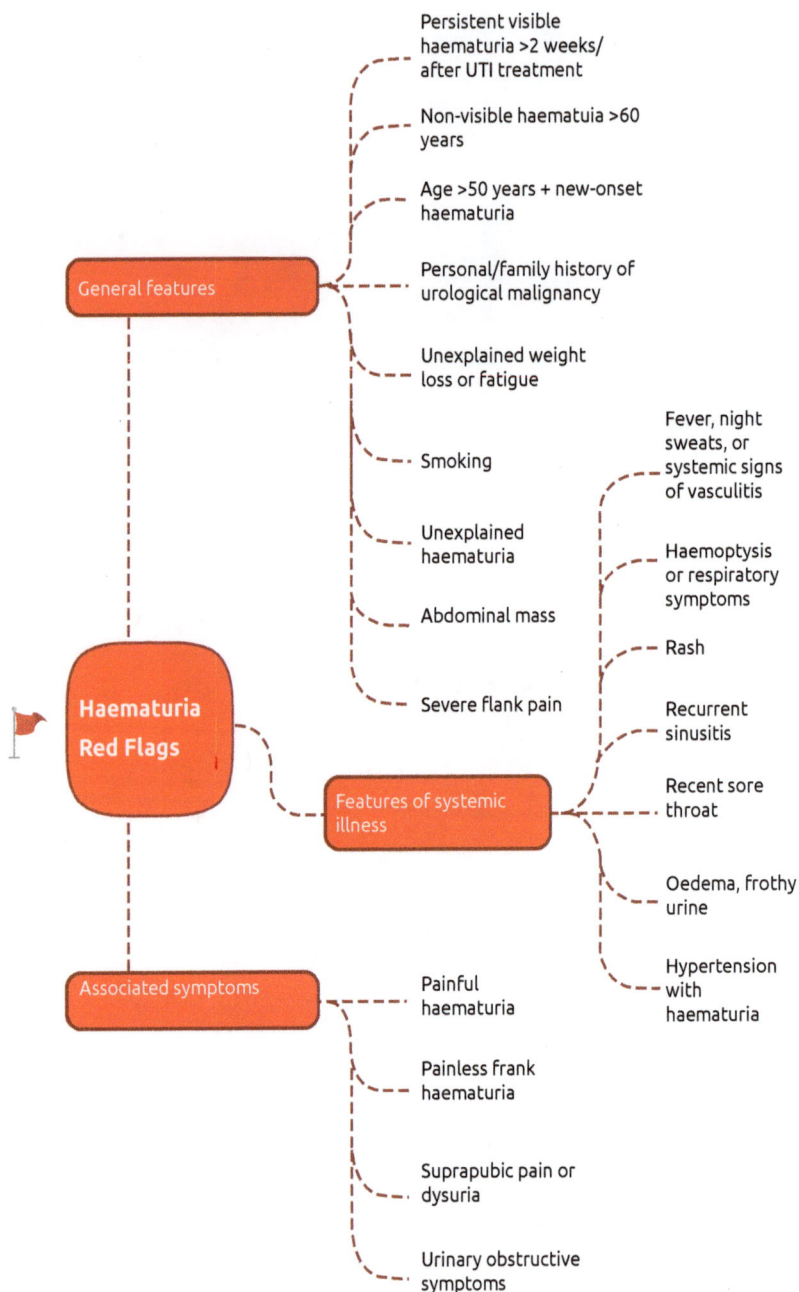

Haematuria Red Flags

General features

- Persistent visible haematuria >2 weeks/ after UTI treatment
- Non-visible haematuia >60 years
- Age >50 years + new-onset haematuria
- Personal/family history of urological malignancy
- Unexplained weight loss or fatigue
- Smoking
- Unexplained haematuria
- Abdominal mass
- Severe flank pain

Features of systemic illness

- Fever, night sweats, or systemic signs of vasculitis
- Haemoptysis or respiratory symptoms
- Rash
- Recurrent sinusitis
- Recent sore throat
- Oedema, frothy urine
- Hypertension with haematuria

Associated symptoms

- Painful haematuria
- Painless frank haematuria
- Suprapubic pain or dysuria
- Urinary obstructive symptoms

History Taking - Important points

1. **DURATION AND TYPE**
- Duration: Is the haematuria recent or long-standing? Chronic haematuria may suggest malignancy or glomerular pathology.
- Type: Is it visible (macroscopic) or non-visible (microscopic)?
- Persistent non-visible haematuria can be associated with glomerular disease or early malignancy.

2. **ASSOCIATED URINARY SYMPTOMS**
- Obstructive Symptoms: Incomplete bladder emptying, nocturia, or difficulty starting/stopping urine flow (suggests prostatic hypertrophy or urethral obstruction).
- Irritative Symptoms: Urgency, frequency, dysuria (consider UTI, bladder cancer, or inflammatory conditions).

3. **PAIN AND LOCATION**
- Flank Pain: Suggests renal calculi, infarction, or obstruction.
- Painless Frank Haematuria: Highly concerning for malignancy.

4. **SYSTEMIC FEATURES**
- Recent sore throat or respiratory symptoms: Could indicate post-streptococcal glomerulonephritis or systemic vasculitis.
- Haemoptysis or cough: Consider Goodpasture's syndrome or ANCA-associated vasculitis (e.g., Wegener's granulomatosis).
- Fever or chills: Possible pyelonephritis or infection.

5. **MEDICAL AND FAMILY HISTORY**
- Personal History: Any known renal disease, nephrotic syndrome, recurrent urinary infections, or trauma (e.g., catheterisation).
- Family History: Renal disease, polycystic kidney disease, or cancer.

6. **LIFESTYLE AND MEDICATIONS**
- Smoking: Increases risk of bladder and renal cancers.
- Occupational exposure: Working with carcinogens like dyes or industrial chemicals.
- Anticoagulants: Raises concern for bleeding disorders or provoked haematuria.

7. **ADDITIONAL CONSIDERATIONS**
- Presence of flank tenderness or a palpable mass (renal cell carcinoma or advanced disease).
- Hypertension: May indicate underlying glomerular disease or renal impairment.
- Proteinuria: A sign of glomerular involvement.
- History of recent infections or systemic inflammatory conditions.

Are you missing something?

- **Bladder cancer:** Particularly in patients >50 years or with a smoking history.
- **Renal cell carcinoma:** Consider in patients with haematuria, flank pain, and a palpable mass.
- **Renal vasculitis:** Suspect with haematuria, systemic signs, and abnormal renal function.
- **Glomerulonephritis:** Look for proteinuria, hypertension, and dysmorphic red cells.

Top tips

CLINICAL PATTERNS TO NOTE
- Painless visible haematuria: Strongly suggests malignancy.
- Painful haematuria: Often caused by stones or infection.
- Proteinuria with haematuria: Suggests glomerular disease.

Diagnostic sieves
■ □ ▨ +

Serious diagnoses to consider

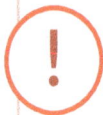

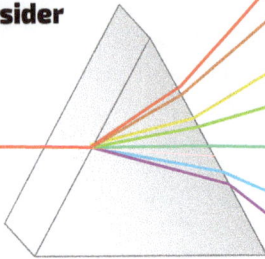

(!)

Bladder Cancer

Renal Cell Carcinoma

Perforated Viscus (e.g. from Peptic Ulcer or Diverticulitis)

Glomerulonephritis

Renal Tuberculosis

Endocarditis

Pyelonephritis

❗ SERIOUS SYMPTOMS!

- Painless frank haematuria is highly concerning for malignancies (ie. **bladder or upper urothelial carcinoma**)
- Persistent irritative symptoms (e.g., frequency, urgency) with haematuria in older adults often suggest **bladder cancer.**
- Flank pain, haematuria, and a palpable mass are indicative of **renal cell carcinoma or polycystic kidney disease.**
- Recurrent visible haematuria following infections suggests **glomerulonephritis or IgA nephropathy.**
- Systemic symptoms such as fever, night sweats, or weight loss raise suspicion for **renal tuberculosis or malignancy.**
- Haematuria with associated rash, joint pain, or fever suggests **systemic vasculitis,** such as **lupus nephritis or granulomatosis with polyangiitis.**

❗ SERIOUS SIGNS!

- Flank tenderness/palpable abdominal mass suggests **renal cell carcinoma or polycystic kidney disease.**
- Proteinuria (particularly significant with haematuria), suggests glomerular disease (ie. **glomerulonephritis, lupus nephritis**).
- Dysmorphic red blood cells/red cell casts on urine microscopy are diagnostic of **glomerular haematuria** (ie. **glomerulonephritis**).
- Signs of renal failure (e.g., elevated creatinine, reduced urine output) & haematuria suggest **advanced kidney disease or severe vasculitis.**
- Hypertension with haematuria is a key feature of **glomerulonephritis or renovascular pathology.**
- Murmurs (e.g., due to **endocarditis**) & haematuria suggest **embolic renal infarction or vasculitis.**
- Visible haematuria with clot retention or obstruction necessitates urgent evaluation for malignancy or structural abnormalities.

- Recurrent haematuria post-infection: Common in IgA nephropathy.
- Red or tea-coloured urine: May indicate glomerular origin

APPROACH TO DIAGNOSIS

Initial evaluation:

- Urinalysis and microscopy (look for red cells, casts, and protein).
- Blood tests: FBC, U&Es, coagulation profile.

Imaging:

Renal ultrasound or CT urography.

Specialist referral:

- Consider urgent urology referral for suspected malignancy.
- Nephrology referral if glomerular disease or systemic vasculitis suspected.

Beware of false haematuria: Certain foods (e.g., beetroot) or medications can mimic haematuria

Differential diagnosis of haematuria

Category	Examples
V – Vascular	Renal infarction, renal vein thrombosis, renal vasculitis.
I – Infectious	Pyelonephritis, urinary tract infection (UTI), renal tuberculosis.
T – Trauma	Blunt or penetrating trauma to the kidney or bladder, post-catheterisation or post-surgical haematuria.
A – Autoimmune	Lupus nephritis, glomerulonephritis (e.g., post-infectious, IgA nephropathy, membranoproliferative).
M – Metabolic	Hypercalcaemia leading to nephrolithiasis.
I – Idiopathic	Essential or idiopathic haematuria (diagnosis of exclusion).
N – Neoplastic	Bladder cancer, renal cell carcinoma, urothelial carcinoma of the upper tract.
D – Degenerative	Benign prostatic hyperplasia (BPH).
C – Congenital	Polycystic kidney disease, congenital vascular malformations.

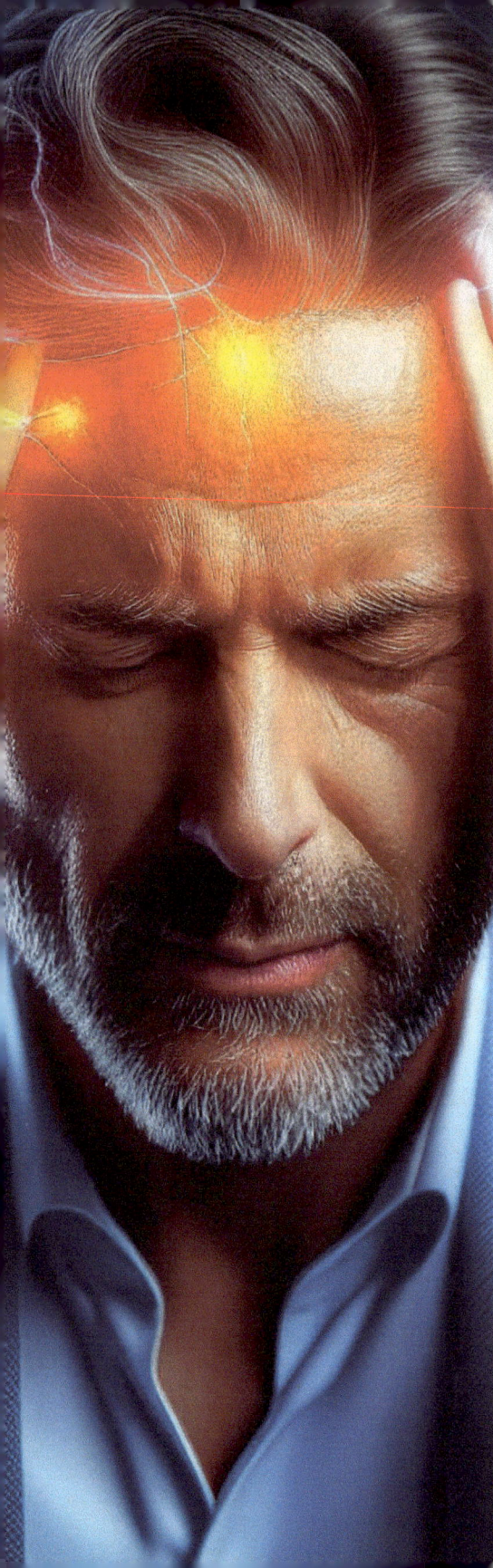

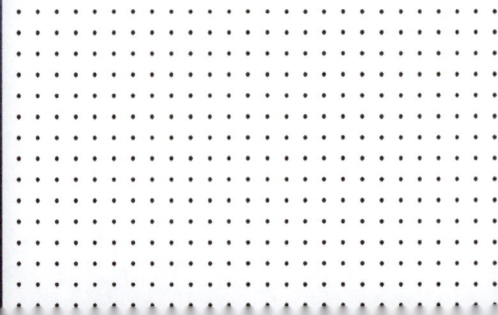

18
Headache

Headaches are one of the most common presenting complaints in both primary care and emergency settings. While many headaches are benign and self-limiting, a thorough evaluation is essential to rule out serious underlying pathology. This chapter highlights the red flags, differential diagnoses, and structured approaches necessary to differentiate between primary and secondary causes of headaches. The "VITA-MIN-C" framework provides a systematic method for categorizing potential causes, enabling clinicians to promptly identify and manage life-threatening conditions.

Diagnostic sieves

Headache Red Flags

History

- Sudden onset severe headache
- New or different headache in a patient >50 years
- Persistent headache despite treatment
- Headache aggravated by coughing, straining, or lying down
- Morning headache with N&V
- Visual disturbances
- New seizure
- Fever or neck stiffness
- Weight loss or night sweats
- IV Drug User
- Headache in third trimester
- History of Cancer
- Immunocompromised
- Recent trauma
- History of neurosurgery
- On blood thinning medications
- Alcohol excess history

Examination

- New focal neurology
- Confusion, drowsiness, or reduced GCS
- Non-blanching rash
- Papilledema
- Scalp tenderness or jaw claudication
- Cranial nerve palsies

History Taking - Important points

1. SITE:
- Where is the pain located?

2. ONSET:
- When did the pain start? Was it sudden or gradual? Is this the first episode?

3. CHARACTERISTICS:
- How does the pain feel (e.g., sharp, dull, aching, burning)?
- Radiates: Does it radiate?

4. ASSOCIATED SYMPTOMS:
- Any visual changes (e.g., blurring, double vision, visual field defects)?
- Neck stiffness? Sensitivity to light or sound?
- Weakness, numbness, or tingling in any limbs?
- Speech or swallowing difficulties?
- Fever, weight loss, night sweats, or fatigue?
- Nausea or vomiting? (especially morning vomiting)
- Runny nose, red or watery eyes?

5. TIMING:
- Is the pain constant, intermittent, or worse at a particular time (e.g. night, morning)?

6. EXACERBATING/RELIEVING FACTORS:
- Does anything trigger the headache? (e.g., stress, sleep deprivation, certain foods, coughing, bending over)
- Does anything make the headache better? (e.g., rest, darkness, medication)

7. SEVERITY:
- How severe is the pain on a scale of 1 to 10?

8. PAST MEDICAL HISTORY:
- Known conditions (e.g., hypertension, cancer, immunosuppression, connective tissue disease)?
- Recent head trauma?

9. MEDICATION HISTORY:
- Current medications (any anticoagulants, oral contraceptives)?
- Overuse of pain medications (risk of medication-overuse headache)?
- Recent steroid withdrawal?

10. FAMILY AND SOCIAL HISTORY:
Family History:
- Family history of migraines or other neurological disorders?

Differential diagnoses using the VITAMIN-C framework

Category	Conditions
Vascular	Subarachnoid hemorrhage, cerebral venous sinus thrombosis (CVST), carotid/vertebral artery dissection, hypertensive crisis.
Infectious	Meningitis, encephalitis, cerebral abscess.
Trauma	Post-traumatic headache.
Autoimmune	Temporal arteritis (giant cell arteritis).
Metabolic	Hypertensive crisis, preeclampsia/eclampsia.
Idiopathic	Medication-overuse headache, benign intracranial hypertension.
Neoplastic	Intracranial space-occupying lesion (SOL), pituitary apoplexy.
Congenital	Chiari malformation.

Diagnostic sieves
■ ☐ ☐ +

Serious diagnoses to consider

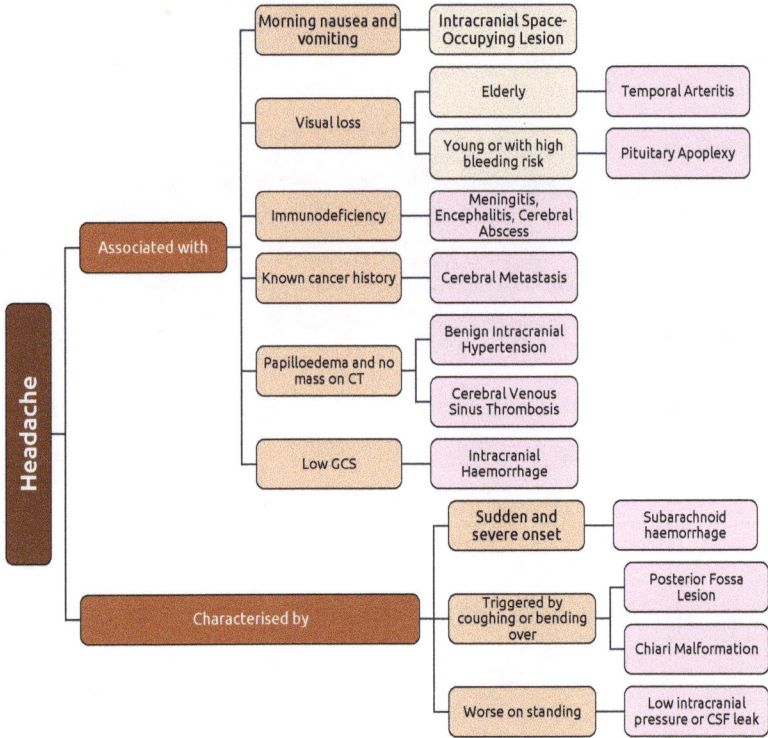

Headache

Associated with

- Morning nausea and vomiting → Intracranial Space-Occupying Lesion
- Visual loss
  - Elderly → Temporal Arteritis
  - Young or with high bleeding risk → Pituitary Apoplexy
- Immunodeficiency → Meningitis, Encephalitis, Cerebral Abscess
- Known cancer history → Cerebral Metastasis
- Papilloedema and no mass on CT
  - Benign Intracranial Hypertension
  - Cerebral Venous Sinus Thrombosis
- Low GCS → Intracranial Haemorrhage

Characterised by

- Sudden and severe onset → Subarachnoid haemorrhage
- Triggered by coughing or bending over
  - Posterior Fossa Lesion
  - Chiari Malformation
- Worse on standing → Low intracranial pressure or CSF leak

ⓘ SERIOUS SYMPTOMS!

- Papilledema: Indicates raised intracranial pressure, often due to intracranial space-occupying lesions or cerebral venous sinus thrombosis.
- Scalp tenderness or jaw claudication: Suggests temporal arteritis, especially in patients over 50 years.
- Non-blanching rash: Raises concern for meningitis or septicemia.
- Cranial nerve palsies: Associated with pituitary apoplexy, intracranial tumors, or cavernous sinus thrombosis.
- Confusion, drowsiness, or reduced GCS: Indicates significant neurological impairment, potentially from intracranial hemorrhage, meningitis, or encephalitis

ⓘ SERIOUS SIGNS!

- Sudden severe "thunderclap" headache: Suggests subarachnoid hemorrhage or carotid/vertebral artery dissection.
- Morning headache with nausea and vomiting: Indicates raised intracranial pressure, commonly from tumors or benign intracranial hypertension.
- Fever and neck stiffness: Point to meningitis or encephalitis.
- Visual disturbances (blurring, field defects): Suggest pituitary apoplexy, temporal arteritis, or raised intracranial pressure.
- Progressive neurological deficits: Raise concerns for brain tumors, cerebral abscess, or strokes involving posterior circulation.
- Weight loss or night sweats: Suggest malignancy, cerebral metastasis, or temporal arteritis.

Social History:
- Stress, lifestyle, sleep patterns, alcohol use, smoking, drug use (e.g., cocaine).

Are you missing something?

Temporal Arteritis (Giant Cell Arteritis): Unilateral headache with scalp tenderness, jaw claudication, and visual disturbances in patients >50 years.

Benign Intracranial Hypertension (BIH): Headache in overweight women, often accompanied by visual disturbances and papilledema.

CRITICAL DIAGNOSES NOT TO MISS

Subarachnoid Hemorrhage: Always consider in patients with sudden, severe headache described as "thunderclap."

Cerebral Venous Sinus Thrombosis (CVST): Headache with focal deficits, seizures, or visual changes, often postpartum or in hypercoagulable states.

Eclampsia: Headache in the third trimester of pregnancy, accompanied by hypertension, proteinuria, or seizures.

Intracranial Space-Occupying Lesion: Persistent, progressive headache with morning nausea/vomiting, focal neurological deficits, and papilledema.

Meningitis: Always evaluate for fever, neck stiffness, and rash, as delayed treatment can be fatal.

Top tips

CHRONIC VS. NEW-ONSET HEADACHES:
- Chronic headaches are typically primary (e.g., migraines, tension headaches).
- New headaches are more likely secondary and require a thorough evaluation.
- A headache identical in quality to chronic headaches is less concerning than a mild headache with a completely new pattern.

Key Signs and Symptoms:
- Headache on waking, worsened by stooping, coughing, or straining suggests raised ICP.
- Headaches without vomiting or visual disturbances are more typical of tension headaches.

Migraine Diagnosis:
- Migraines and tension headaches account for 90% of headaches in primary care (https://pmc.ncbi.nlm.nih.gov/articles/PMC4590146/#:~:text=Migraine%20and%20tension%2Dtype%20headaches,to%20primary%20or%20secondary%20care.) Auras (e.g., zigzags, flashes) with migraines are common and typically last ~20 minutes.
- Avoid diagnosing migraine in patients >40 without excluding more serious conditions.

Examination key considerations

Vital Signs:
- Blood pressure (hypertension may indicate malignant hypertension or preeclampsia).
- Temperature (to check for fever suggesting infection).
- Heart rate (tachycardia in sepsis, bradycardia with raised ICP).

Head and Neck Examination:
- Palpation:
  - Tenderness over sinuses (sinusitis).
  - Scalp tenderness (temporal arteritis).
- Neck:
  - Assess for neck stiffness (meningitis, subarachnoid hemorrhage).

Neurological Examination:
- Cranial Nerves:
  - Visual fields, acuity, and fundoscopic exam (look for papilloedema or optic neuritis).
  - Extraocular movements (cranial nerve palsies, e.g., III, IV, VI).

- Facial sensation and symmetry.

Motor and Sensory:

- Limb weakness or sensory deficits.

Cerebellar Exam:

- Check for ataxia, nystagmus, and coordination issues.

Reflexes:

- Hyperreflexia or asymmetry may suggest a space-occupying lesion.

Fundoscopy:

- Look for:
  - Papilloedema (raised ICP).
  - Optic atrophy or hemorrhages.

Gait Assessment:

- Assess for unsteadiness (cerebellar or vestibular dysfunction).

Additional Specific Examinations:

- Temporal Arteries:
  - Check for thickening, tenderness, or absent pulsation (temporal arteritis).
- Jaw Claudication:
  - Ask if chewing causes pain (temporal arteritis).

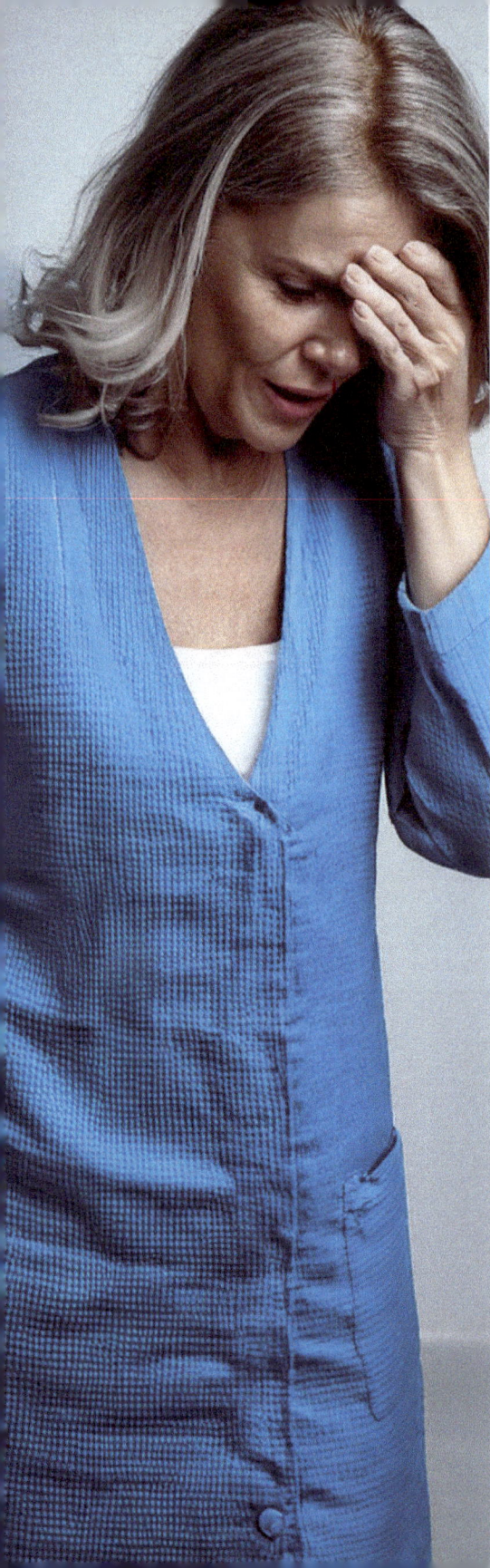

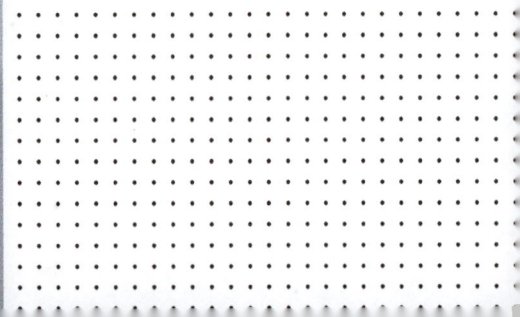

19
Dizziness

Dizziness is a complex symptom that encompasses a wide spectrum of sensations, including lightheadedness, vertigo, disequilibrium, and presyncope. It can originate from a variety of systems, including the neurological, cardiovascular, vestibular, or systemic. While many causes are benign, dizziness can also indicate serious underlying conditions such as stroke, arrhythmias, or intracranial hemorrhage. Accurate diagnosis hinges on detailed history-taking, physical examination, and targeted investigations to distinguish between peripheral and central causes and to identify red flags that necessitate urgent intervention.

Diagnostic sieves

Dizziness Red Flags

Severe symptoms
- Severe headache, especially sudden or "thunderclap"
- Altered consciousness or confusion
- Persistent dizziness with chest pain or palpitations

Neurological deficits
- New gait abnormalities or ataxia
- Focal neurological deficits (e.g., weakness, numbness, dysarthria)

Cardiovascular concerns
- Arrhythmias causing dizziness or syncope
- Family history of sudden cardiac death or known arrhythmias

Recent history or events
- Recent head trauma or neck injury
- Recent infection (e.g., upper respiratory tract infection, sinusitis)

Differential diagnosis of dizziness

Category	Examples
V – Vascular	Stroke, transient ischemic attack (TIA), intracranial hemorrhage, carotid or vertebral artery dissection.
I – Infectious	Vestibular neuritis, labyrinthitis, meningitis, encephalitis.
T – Trauma	Post-concussion syndrome, traumatic brain injury, labyrinthine concussion.
A – Autoimmune	Multiple sclerosis, autoimmune inner ear disease (AIED), vasculitis (e.g., polyarteritis nodosa).
M – Metabolic	Electrolyte imbalances (e.g., hyponatremia, hypoglycemia), anemia, hypercalcemia.
I – Idiopathic	Persistent postural-perceptual dizziness (PPPD), idiopathic vertigo.
N – Neoplastic	Brain tumors, acoustic neuroma (vestibular schwannoma), cerebellopontine angle tumors.
D – Degenerative	Degenerative cervical spine disease causing vertebrobasilar insufficiency.
C – Congenital	Arnold-Chiari malformation, congenital vestibular dysfunction.

History Taking - Important points

1. ONSET

- Sudden onset: Suggests stroke, TIA, vertebral or carotid artery dissection, arrhythmias, or cardiac ischemia.
- Gradual onset: Indicates brain tumors, multiple sclerosis, or metabolic imbalances like anemia.

2. NATURE

- Spinning sensation (vertigo): Likely vestibular causes (e.g., post-traumatic vertigo, cerebellopontine lesions).
- Lightheadedness: Suggests hypoglycemia, anemia, arrhythmias, or aortic stenosis.
- Sense of imbalance: May indicate brain tumor, cerebellar lesions, or multiple sclerosis.

3. TRIGGERS

- Exertion: Points to cardiac ischemia or aortic stenosis.
- Head movements or posture changes: Associated with post-traumatic vertigo or vestibular issues.
- Hyperventilation: Suggests anxiety-related dizziness or functional causes.

4. DURATION AND FREQUENCY

- Seconds to minutes: TIA, arrhythmias, or anxiety-related dizziness.
- Minutes to hours: Vertebral artery dissection, metabolic imbalances, or functional causes.

- Recurrent episodes: Multiple sclerosis, arrhythmias, or anxiety.

5. ASSOCIATED SYMPTOMS

Neurological Symptoms:

- Weakness, numbness, or speech changes: Stroke, TIA, or multiple sclerosis.
- Visual disturbances: Vertebral or carotid artery dissection, brain tumor.

Infectious Symptoms:

- Fever, neck stiffness, or altered mental status: Intracranial abscess or meningitis.

Cardiac Symptoms:

- Chest pain or palpitations: Arrhythmias or cardiac ischemia.
- Syncope or dyspnea: Aortic stenosis or arrhythmias.

Other Symptoms:

- Fatigue, pallor: Severe anemia.
- Diaphoresis, irritability: Hypoglycemia.

6. ILLNESS AND MEDICATION HISTORY

- Recent Infections: Suggests meningitis, intracranial abscess, or post-viral dizziness.
- Trauma: Points to concussion or vertebral artery dissection.
- New Medications or Dose Changes: May cause dizziness due to side effects (e.g., antihypertensives, sedatives).

Are you missing something?

- **Posterior Circulation Stroke:** Sudden vertigo with focal signs (e.g., ataxia, visual changes).
- **Arrhythmias:** Lightheadedness with syncope or chest pain.
- **Vertebral artery dissection:** consider if neck pain present

Always consider stroke in patients with sudden vertigo and neurological deficits.

Suspect arrhythmias in patients with dizziness and syncope.

Rule out carotid or vertebral artery dissection in trauma patients with dizziness and neck pain.

Top tips

- Differentiate vertigo (spinning sensation) from dizziness (lightheadedness).
- Don't overlook systemic causes like anemia or metabolic imbalances.

Serious diagnoses to consider

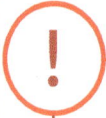

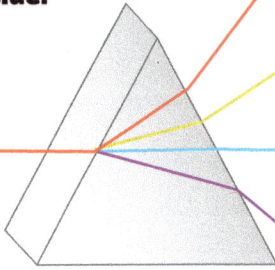

Stroke or TIA:
Sudden onset dizziness with focal neurological signs like hemiparesis or dysarthria.

Cardiac Arrhythmias:
Dizziness due to cerebral hypoperfusion from bradycardia or atrial fibrillation.

Vertebral or Carotid Artery Dissection:
Dizziness with neck pain, often post-trauma.

Labyrinthitis or Vestibular Neuritis:
Persistent vertigo with nausea and vomiting, often post-viral infection.

! SERIOUS SYMPTOMS!

- Sudden onset weakness or numbness.
- Hearing loss or tinnitus.
- Severe nausea or vomiting unresponsive to treatment.
- Persistent vertigo with functional impairment.

! SERIOUS SIGNS!

- Focal neurological deficits (e.g. weakness, speech difficulty).
- Vertical or direction-changing nystagmus.
- Gait ataxia or unsteadiness.
- Severe headache or auditory symptoms like unilateral tinnitus

- Always assess for auditory and neurological symptoms to exclude central causes.
- postural hypotension is not always a benign diagnosis, consider chronic causes of postural hypotension such as polypharmacy, heart failure, Addisons disease etc.
- it's often worth noting patients don't clearly describe or differentiate between the above sensations (vertigo, pre-syncope etc) so keep your differentials broad and exclude red flags
- Ask about her nature of the dizziness
- Avoid putting words into the patient's mouth
- It is likely the answer will fall into one of the 4 categories which are: (see diagram below)

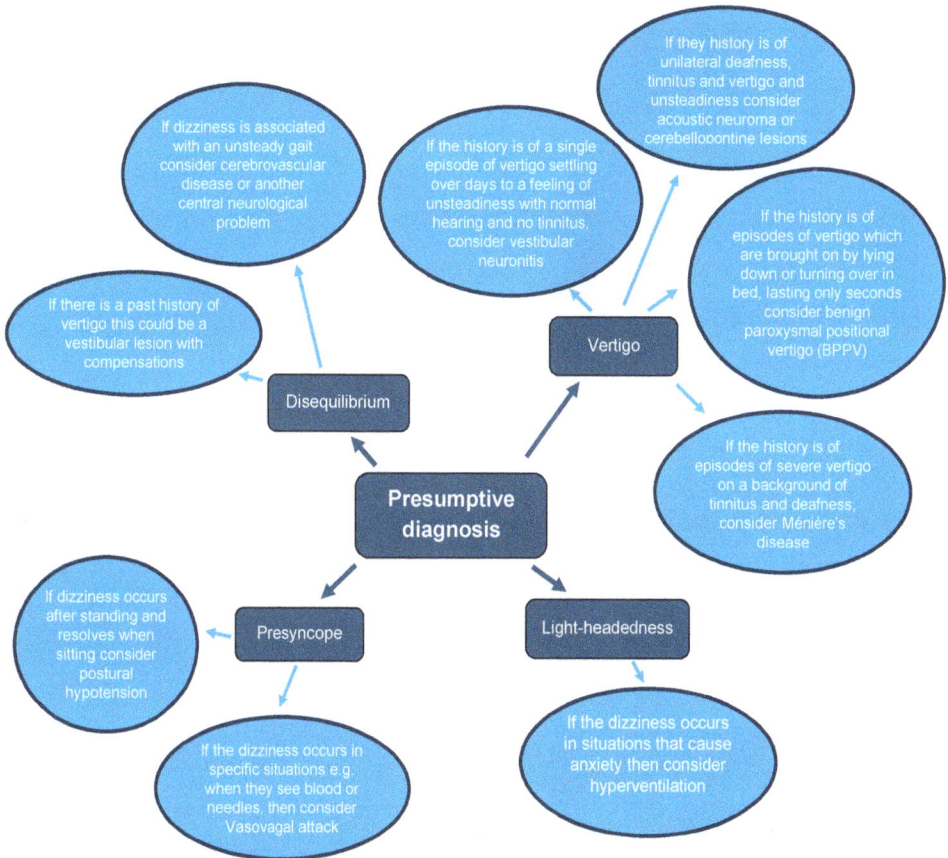

If they history is of unilateral deafness, tinnitus and vertigo and unsteadiness consider acoustic neuroma or cerebellopontine lesions

If dizziness is associated with an unsteady gait consider cerebrovascular disease or another central neurological problem

If the history is of a single episode of vertigo settling over days to a feeling of unsteadiness with normal hearing and no tinnitus, consider vestibular neuronitis

If the history is of episodes of vertigo which are brought on by lying down or turning over in bed, lasting only seconds consider benign paroxysmal positional vertigo (BPPV)

If there is a past history of vertigo this could be a vestibular lesion with compensations

Disequilibrium

Vertigo

Presumptive diagnosis

If the history is of episodes of severe vertigo on a background of tinnitus and deafness, consider Méniére's disease

If dizziness occurs after standing and resolves when sitting consider postural hypotension

Presyncope

Light-headedness

If the dizziness occurs in specific situations e.g. when they see blood or needles, then consider Vasovagal attack

If the dizziness occurs in situations that cause anxiety then consider hyperventilation

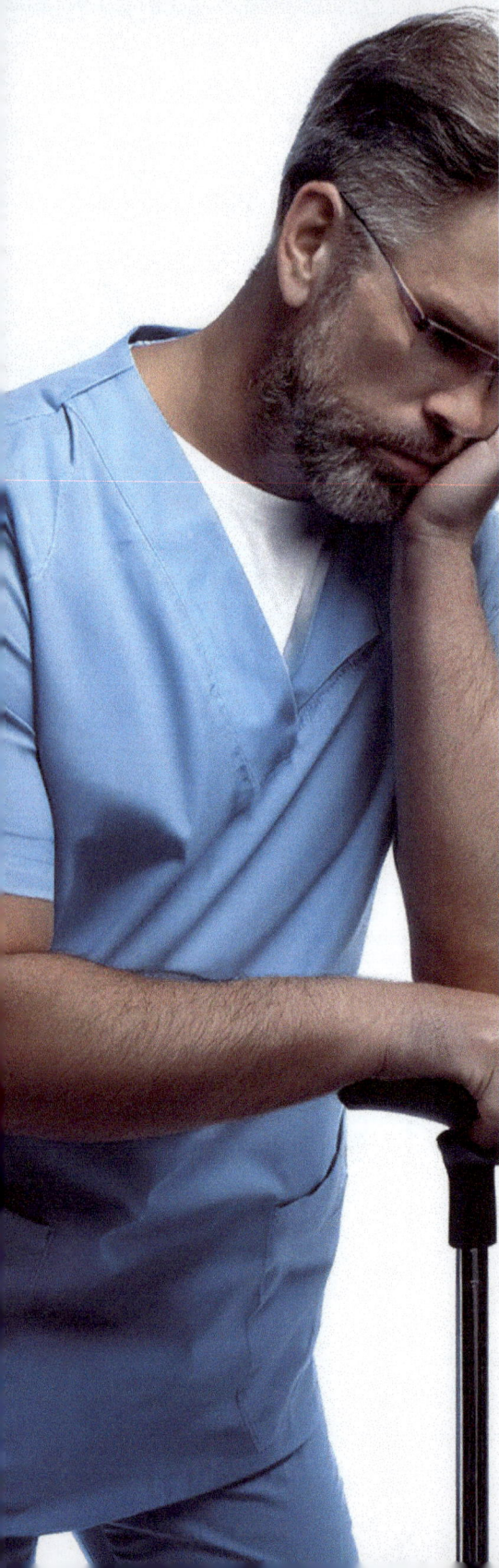

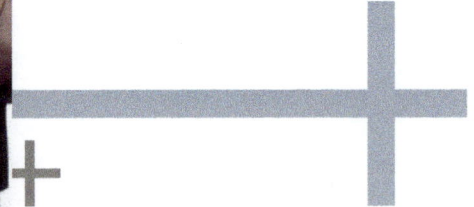

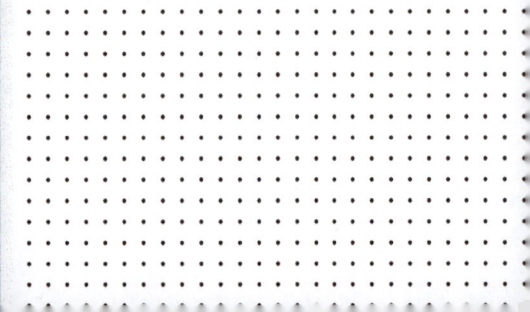

20
Vertigo

Vertigo is a specific type of dizziness characterized by a false sense of spinning or movement, either of oneself or the surroundings. It is a common yet disconcerting symptom with causes ranging from benign peripheral conditions, such as benign paroxysmal positional vertigo (BPPV), to serious central pathologies like posterior circulation strokes. Understanding the nuances of vertigo presentation, alongside targeted investigations, is key to effective diagnosis and management.

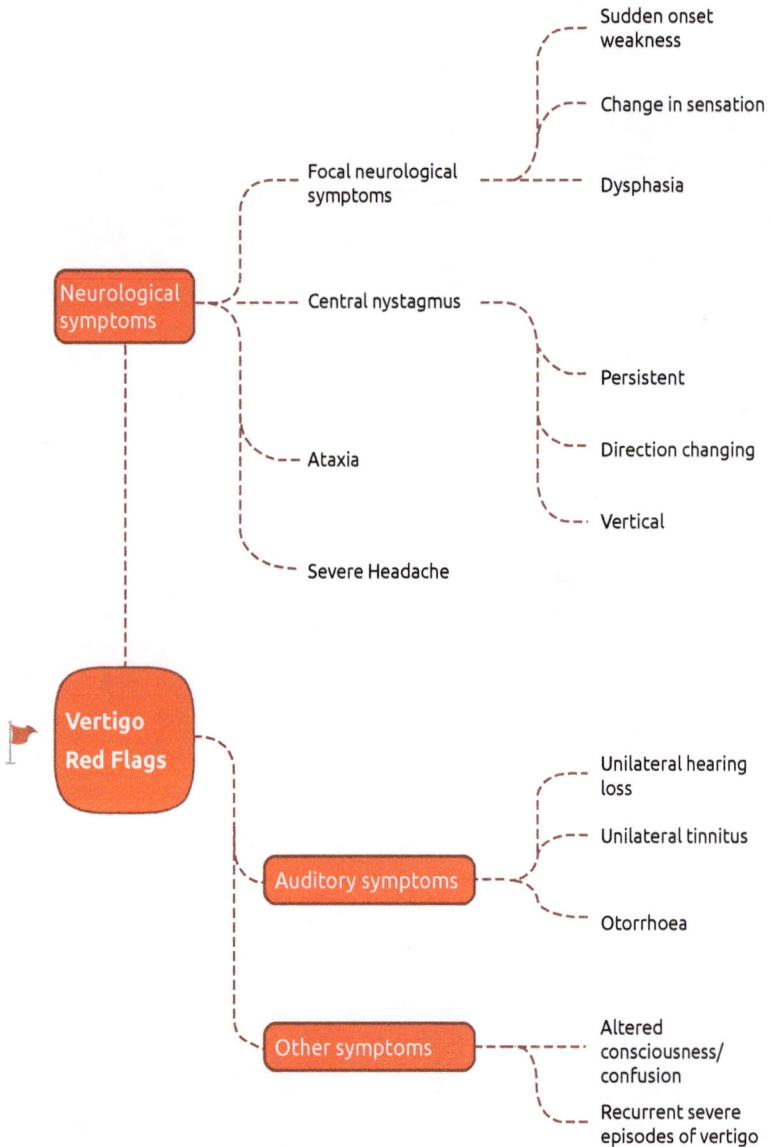

Neurological symptoms

Focal neurological symptoms
- Sudden onset weakness
- Change in sensation
- Dysphasia

Central nystagmus
- Persistent
- Direction changing
- Vertical

Ataxia

Severe Headache

Vertigo Red Flags

Auditory symptoms
- Unilateral hearing loss
- Unilateral tinnitus
- Otorrhoea

Other symptoms
- Altered consciousness/ confusion
- Recurrent severe episodes of vertigo

History Taking - Important points

Was the vertigo sudden or gradual in onset?

- Sudden: Suggests BPPV, acute labyrinthitis, acute vestibular neuritis, or posterior circulation stroke.
- Gradual: Suggests Meniere's disease, vestibular migraine, or a central cause like a tumor (e.g., Acoustic Neuroma, Brainstem Tumor).

How long do the symptoms last (seconds, minutes, hours, or days)?

- Seconds to minutes: BPPV.
- Minutes to Hours: Meniere's disease, Vestibular migraine

- Hours to days: Acute vestibular neuritis, labyrinthitis
- Recurrent or persistent: Acoustic neuroma, multiple sclerosis (MS), brainstem tumour

What brings on the symptoms (head movement, standing up, or lying down)?

- Position changes: Suggest BPPV.
- Standing up: Orthostatic hypotension* Link to top tip
- No clear trigger: Central causes or Meniere's disease

Examination

HEAD IMPULSE NYSTAGMUS TEST OF SKEW (HINTS) EXAM

Peripheral causes: Abnormal head impulse test, unidirectional horizontal nystagmus, no skew deviation.

Central causes: Normal head impulse test, bidirectional or vertical nystagmus, skew deviation.

DIX-HALLPIKE MANEUVER- TESTS FOR BENIGN PAROXYSMAL POSITIONAL VERITGO

Positive: Vertigo and torsional nystagmus triggered by positional changes, resolving within a minute.

CRANIAL NERVE EXAMINATION

Focus on cranial nerves II, III, IV, VI, and VIII.

Diplopia, nystagmus, or gaze palsies suggest central lesions (brainstem or cerebellum).

Hearing loss or tinnitus may indicate Meniere's disease or labyrinthitis.

Key considerations

CT scans have low sensitivity for identifying acute infarcts, particularly in the posterior fossa.

MRI is not always available and may produce false-negative results in early acute posterior circulation strokes.

This highlights the importance of history and examination in making an effective diagnosis for vertigo!

VERTIGO VS DIZZINESS

Dizziness is a broad term describing sensations of lightheadedness, faintness, or unsteadiness, often caused by low blood pressure, dehydration, or anxiety. It can also result from various cardiovascular, neurological, or vestibular issues.

Vertigo, however, is a specific type of dizziness characterized by the sensation of spinning, usually due to disorders of the inner ear or brainstem.

While vertigo often points to a vestibular problem, dizziness can stem from a wider array of causes

Diagnostic sieves

⚠ SERIOUS SYMPTOMS!

Neurological symptoms

- Focal neurological deficits: such as sudden-onset weakness, numbness, or speech difficulties, which could indicate a stroke.
- Central nystagmus: Persistent, direction-changing, or vertical nystagmus, suggestive of brainstem or cerebellar pathology.
- Ataxia or unsteady gait: New or worsening gait disturbance suggests cerebellar or brainstem dysfunction. Often associated with a posterior circulation stroke.
- Severe headache: Accompanied by neurological symptoms, potentially indicative of posterior circulation stroke or other central causes

Auditory symptoms

- Unilateral hearing loss or tinnitus: May point to conditions such as vestibular schwannoma or labyrinthine infarction.
- Otorrhoea (ear discharge): Could indicate infection or endolymphatic fistula

Other

- Altered consciousness/confusion: Could indicate seizures, stroke or serious cardiac causes
- Recurrent, severe episodes of vertigo: Especially if unresponsive to treatment or associated with significant functional impairment

Top tips

Postural Hypotension Considerations:

- Chronic causes include polypharmacy, Addison's disease, and autonomic dysfunction.

Broaden the Differential:

- Patients often struggle to describe the nature of dizziness; exclude serious causes (stroke, arrhythmia).

Central Red Flags:

- Vertigo with focal neurological signs or central nystagmus should prompt imaging.

Peripheral vs. Central:

- Use HINTS testing in acute, continuous vertigo to differentiate peripheral from central causes.

Differential diagnosis of Vertigo

	Cause	Key features	Findings	Associated Symptoms
Peripheral causes of vertigo	Benign Paroxysmal Positional Vertigo (BPPV)	Sudden, brief episodes (seconds to minutes) triggered by head movements.	Positive Dix-Hallpike manoeuvre; torsional nystagmus	No hearing loss or tinnitus. Episodes are isolated to vertigo without systemic symptoms.
	Acute Vestibular Neuritis	Sudden-onset vertigo lasting days with nausea and vomiting. Typically follows a viral infection.	Unidirectional nystagmus; impaired head impulse test	No hearing loss or tinnitus
	Labyrinthitis	Vertigo lasting days, often following a viral infection. Similar to vestibular neuritis but includes hearing loss or tinnitus.	Unidirectional nystagmus with auditory deficits (sensorineural hearing loss on audiometry).	Sudden unilateral hearing loss and tinnitus
	Meniere's Disease	Recurrent, episodic vertigo lasting hours to days.	Progressive sensorineural hearing loss (initially unilateral though can progress to bilateral)	Associated with aural fullness, progressive hearing loss and tinnitus.
	Acoustic Neuroma (Vestibular Schwannoma)	Gradual-onset vertigo, often mild	Unilateral hearing loss in audiometry. Absent corneal reflex or facial nerve palsy in advanced cases.	Slowly progressive hearing loss and sometimes tinnitus.
Central causes of vertigo	Posterior circulation stroke	Sudden, persistent vertigo with focal neurological signs.	Gait ataxia, dysarthria, dysphagia, or hemiparesis. Vertical or direction-changing nystagmus.	Severe headache, diplopia, and limb ataxia. May mimic vestibular neuritis but with red flags like dysmetria.
	Vestibular Migraine	Episodic vertigo associated with migraine features.	Normal neurological exam between episodes	Aura, photophobia, phonophobia
	Multiple Sclerosis (MS)	Gradual or episodic vertigo	Hyperreflexia, weakness, or visual disturbances. MRI may show demyelinating lesions.	Transient visual changes (e.g. optic neuritis), diplopia or paresthesia
	Brainstem Tumours	Gradual-onset vertigo with progressive neurological signs	Diplopia, ataxia, or cranial nerve deficits	Persistent imbalance and progressive gait disturbances.
Systemic or Secondary causes	Orthostatic Hypotension	Dizziness that is often reported as "vertigo" when standing up	Drop in systolic BP >20 mmHg on standing	Lightheadedness or syncope

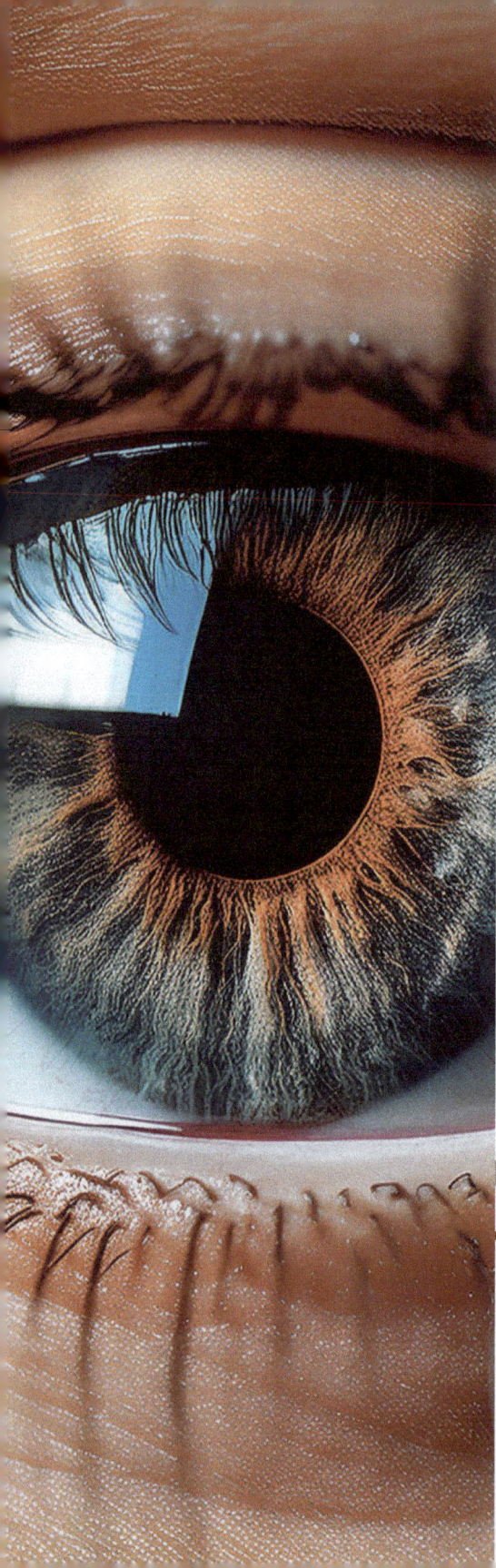

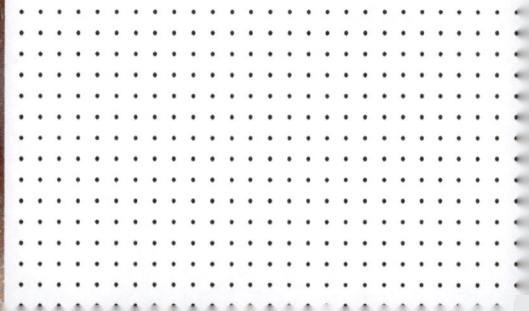

21

Double Vision

Double vision, or **diplopia**, is a significant clinical symptom that requires careful evaluation to determine its underlying cause. It can arise from ocular misalignment, neurological deficits, or systemic diseases. Recognizing red flags, performing a detailed history and examination, and understanding the associated serious diagnoses are crucial to ensure timely diagnosis and management.

Diagnostic sieves

Double Vision Red Flags

- Sudden onset diplopia
- Painful diplopia
- Associated ptosis
- Severe or persistent headache
- Nausea and vomiting
- New anisocoria
- Visual loss
- Worsening/fluctuating diplopia
- Recent facial trauma
- Recent sinusitis or upper respiratory tract infection
- Constitutional symptoms
- New neurological symptoms: weakness, numbness, dysphasia, or altered consciousness

History Taking - Important points

1. NATURE OF DOUBLE VISION:
- Horizontal (medial/lateral rectus), vertical (superior/inferior rectus or oblique muscles), or diagonal.

2. FIELD OF GAZE:
- Which direction worsens diplopia? The worst gaze position often indicates the affected muscle's action field. However, in restrictive disorders (e.g. thyroid eye disease) worsen diplopia opposite to the restricted muscle's primary action.
- In which direction are the images closest? helps differentiate between paretic pathology (caused by weakness or paralysis of an extraocular muscle) and restrictive pathology (caused by mechanical restriction of eye movement). In paretic pathology, the misalignment usually worsens in the direction of action of the weak muscle, while in restrictive pathology, the misalignment often remains consistent or worsens in the opposite direction to the restricted muscle's primary action.

3. PAIN:
- Localised eye pain (orbital cellulitis, inflammation, orbital mass), headache (aneurysm or haemorrhage), trigeminal distribution (intracranial or cavernous sinus lesion)

4. PROGRESSION:
What is the onset, duration, and progression of symptoms?
- Sudden onset: Stroke, aneurysm, trauma.
- Gradual onset: Thyroid eye disease, myasthenia gravis, or neoplastic cause.
- Intermittent symptoms: Myasthenia gravis or fatigue-related disorders.
- Progressive worsening:
- Tumors, inflammation, or degenerative conditions.

5. ASSOCIATED NEUROLOGICAL SYMP-TOMS:
Are there any other neurological symptoms?
- Vision loss or field defects -> Optic nerve involvement.
- Facial numbness or pain ->Trigeminal nerve involvement (cavernous sinus syndrome).
- Hearing loss, dizziness, or imbalance -> Brainstem or cerebellar pathology.
- Dysphagia or speech difficulty -> Brainstem or cranial nerve IX/X dysfunction.
- Ataxia or coordination issues -> Cerebellar lesions.

6. MEDICAL HISTORY:
- Previous migraines, autoimmune diseases, thyroid dysfunction, recent infections, or ocular history (lazy eye/amblyopia, childhood patches or eye surgery, longstanding abnormal head position)

Examination

VISUAL ACUITY
- Test each eye with a Snellen chart, and assess for improvement with a pinhole test.
- Monocular diplopia improving with pinhole indicates refractive error.

PUPILLARY EXAMINATION
Size and reaction:
- Fixed, dilated pupil: Compressive third nerve lesion.
- RAPD: Optic nerve involvement.

Anisocoria:
- Small pupil + ptosis: Horner's syndrome.
- Large pupil + ptosis: Third nerve palsy.

EXTRAOCULAR MOVEMENTS (EOMS)
- Assess ductions and versions in all gaze directions.

Serious diagnoses to consider

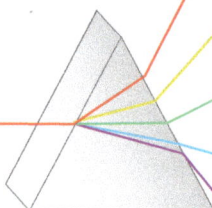

Stroke (Posterior Circulation):
Sudden onset diplopia with neurological deficits like ataxia or dysarthria.

Intracranial Aneurysm:
Painful third nerve palsy, severe headache.

Multiple Sclerosis:
Diplopia from internuclear ophthalmoplegia or optic neuritis.

Myasthenia Gravis:
Intermittent diplopia and ptosis worsening with fatigue.

Cavernous Sinus Thrombosis:
Painful ophthalmoplegia with fever and cranial nerve involvement

! SERIOUS SYMPTOMS!

- Diplopia with severe headache or altered consciousness suggests aneurysm or stroke.
- Fever with diplopia and proptosis suggests orbital cellulitis or cavernous sinus thrombosis.
- Gradual onset with vision changes may indicate thyroid eye disease or intracranial tumor.

! SERIOUS SIGNS!

- Fixed, dilated pupil (compressive third nerve lesion or aneurysm).
- Proptosis and restricted eye movement (orbital cellulitis or tumor).
- Papilledema on fundoscopy (raised intracranial pressure).
- Cranial nerve deficits or facial weakness (brainstem lesions or cavernous sinus pathology).

Double vision differentials using the VITAMIN-C framework

Category	Conditions
V - Vascular	Stroke, intracranial aneurysm, cavernous sinus thrombosis
I - Infectious	Orbital cellulitis, meningitis
T - Trauma	Orbital fracture, post-trauma cranial nerve palsy
A - Autoimmune	Multiple sclerosis, myasthenia gravis
M - Metabolic	Thyroid eye disease
I - Idiopathic	Idiopathic intracranial hypertension, Guillain-Barré syndrome (Miller Fisher variant with ophthalmoplegia)
N - Neoplastic	Brain tumors, orbital tumors
C - Congenital	Congenital strabismus

Identify:
- Comitant diplopia: Misalignment magnitude consistent across gaze (e.g., congenital).
- Incomitant diplopia: Misalignment varies with gaze (e.g., cranial nerve palsies, restrictive disease).

Perform the cover-uncover test:
- Detects tropias (manifest misalignment).

SPECIALIZED TESTS
Three-Step Test (for vertical diplopia):
- Identify hypertropic eye.
- Determine which gaze worsens diplopia.
- Assess head tilt that exacerbates symptoms (implicates specific extraocular muscles).

CRANIAL NERVE EXAMINATION

Check:
- Optic nerve: Visual acuity, color vision, and fields.
- Trigeminal nerve: Facial sensation.
- Facial nerve: Symmetry and strength.
- Vestibulocochlear nerve: Hearing loss or vertigo.

FUNDOSCOPY
Look for:
- Papilledema: Raised intracranial pressure.
- Optic atrophy: Chronic optic neuropathy.
- Retinal pathology or vascular changes.

GLOBE EXAMINATION
Assess for proptosis or displacement:
- Suggests orbital mass or thyroid orbitopathy.
- If available use a Hertel exophthalmometer if proptosis is suspected.

Tips for Diagnostic Localisation

SUPRANUCLEAR CAUSES:
- Vertical or horizontal gaze palsy without alignment changes in the vestibulo-ocular reflex.

NUCLEAR OR INFRANUCLEAR CAUSES:
- Paretic EOMs with corresponding cranial nerve involvement.

RESTRICTIVE CAUSES:
- Limited movement in specific directions with increased intraocular pressure.

CRANIAL NERVE EXAMINATION
- Assess other cranial nerves for:
- Numbness (trigeminal nerve).
- Weakness (facial nerve).
- Hearing loss or ataxia (vestibulocochlear nerve).
- Relevance: Identifies broader cranial

nerve involvement (e.g., cavernous sinus thrombosis).

Are you missing something?

- **Thyroid Eye Disease:** Proptosis, restricted eye movements, and lid retraction.
- **Orbital Cellulitis:** Painful diplopia, swelling, and fever.
- **Idiopathic Intracranial Hypertension:** Sixth nerve palsy, transient visual loss, papilledema.
- **Giant Cell Arteritis:** Vision loss, jaw claudication, scalp tenderness in older patients.

Always consider stroke in patients with diplopia and focal neurological deficits.

Rule out posterior communicating artery aneurysm in painful third nerve palsy.

Suspect cavernous sinus thrombosis in patients with fever, proptosis, and cranial nerve involvement.

Top tips

- Distinguish between monocular (refractive error) and binocular diplopia (neurological or muscular causes).
- Evaluate for systemic symptoms like fever or weight loss to identify systemic diseases.
- MRI is preferred for brain or orbital lesions; CT angiography for suspected aneurysm or sinus thrombosis.
- Review old photographs to identify prior signs of strabismus, ptosis, or misalignment

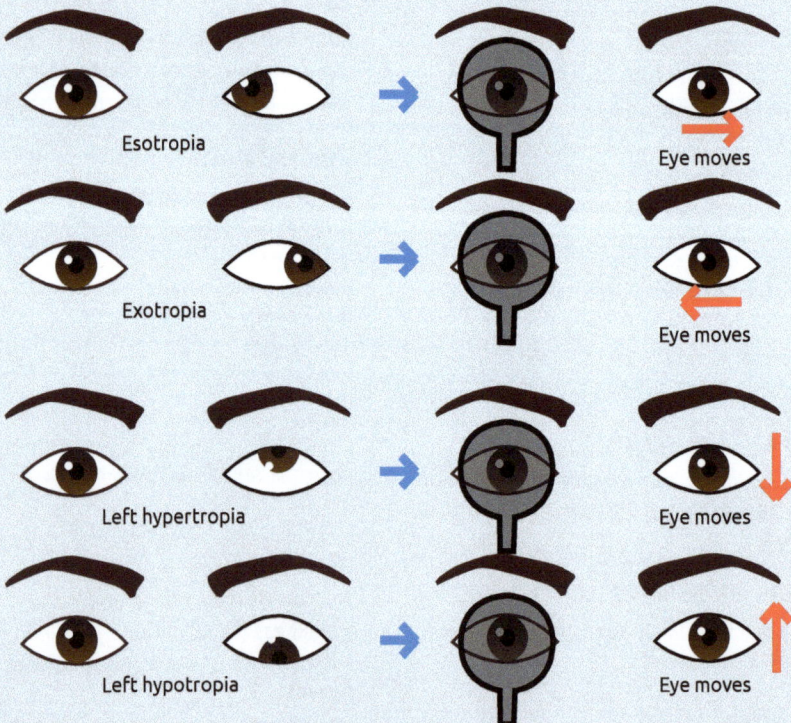

Cover test

Esotropia — Eye moves

Exotropia — Eye moves

Left hypertropia — Eye moves

Left hypotropia — Eye moves

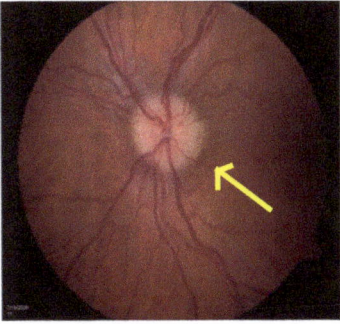

Figure 12.1: Blurred optic disc margin (yellow arrow)
https://eyewiki.org/Papilledema

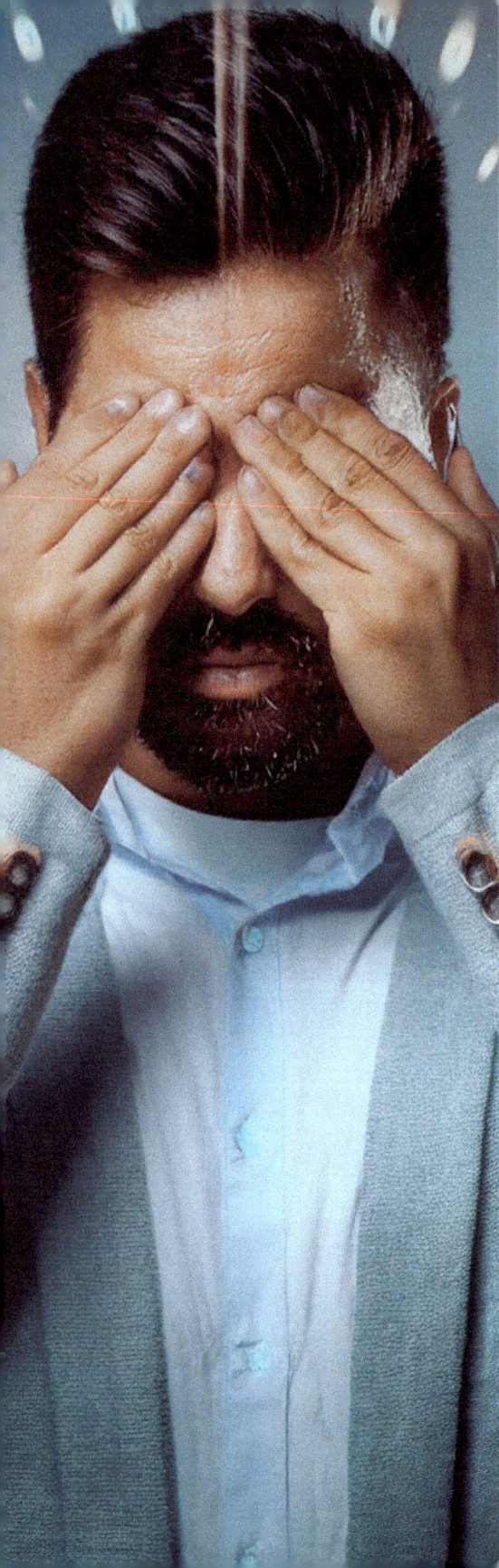

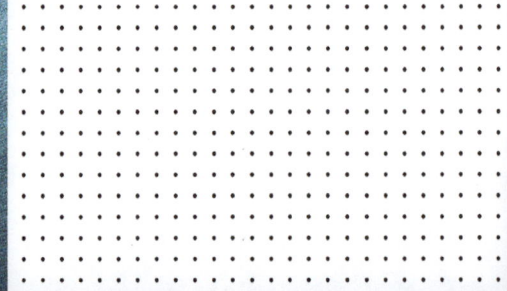

22

Sudden Vision Loss

■ **Sudden vision loss** is an alarming symptom that often signifies a critical underlying condition requiring prompt evaluation. It may arise from vascular, neurological, or ocular pathologies, and differentiating the cause is essential for timely intervention. Whether painful or painless, vision loss—particularly when accompanied by other systemic or ocular symptoms—warrants thorough investigation to rule out life-threatening diagnoses such as stroke, retinal artery occlusion, or acute angle-closure glaucoma.

Vision Loss Red Flags

- Painful loss of vision.

- Visual field loss, even if vision has partially returned.

- Flashes of light, floaters, or a "curtain" effect.

- Red eye, severe headache, or jaw pain.

- Neurological symptoms like confusion or speech difficulty.

- Ocular trauma or history of eye surgery.

- Vascular risk factors: hypertension, diabetes, smoking, atrial fibrillation, thrombophilia.

History Taking - Important points

1. ONSET AND NATURE OF VISION LOSS
- Can you describe when and how the vision loss started? Was it sudden or gradual?
- How long has it lasted so far? Has it improved, worsened, or stayed the same?

2. VISUAL CHARACTERISTICS
- Is the vision loss affecting one eye or both? (Monocular or binocular?)
- Does it involve your entire field of vision, or just a specific part (e.g. central, peripheral, or a specific quadrant)? Looking at my nose with each eye, are any parts of my face missing?
- Have you noticed any patterns, such as a "curtain" effect or shadows?

3. ASSOCIATED EYE SYMPTOMS
- Do you have any eye pain? If yes:
- Is the pain constant, or does it occur with eye movement?
- Have you experienced any other symptoms like flashing lights, floaters, halos around lights, or dark spots (scotomas)?
- Any double vision?

4. SYSTEMIC SYMPTOMS
- Have you noticed any headaches, particularly in your temples? Any scalp tenderness or pain while chewing (jaw claudication)?
- Do you have pain or stiffness in your shoulders or hips (proximal muscle pain)?
- Have you felt sick, had a fever, or experienced fatigue?

5. PAST MEDICAL AND OCULAR HISTORY
- Do you have any history of migraines, especially ones associated with visual symptoms (ocular migraines)?
- Do you have diabetes, high blood pressure, or other cardiovascular conditions? Have you ever had a stroke or transient ischemic attack (TIA)?
- Have you experienced any recent trauma to your eyes or head?
- Do you wear glasses or contact lenses? Any previous eye conditions, surgeries, or treatments?

Are you missing somthing?

- **Amaurosis Fugax:** Transient monocular blindness, warning sign for stroke or embolic event.
- **Retinal Detachment:** Flashes, floaters, and shadow or curtain descending over vision.
- **Vitreous Hemorrhage:** Sudden floaters, diminished red reflex.
- **Non-Arteritic Ischemic Optic Neuropathy:** Monocular vision loss on waking, swollen optic nerve.

Always suspect stroke in patients with sudden vision loss and focal neurological signs.

Rule out Giant Cell Arteritis in patients over 50 with headache, jaw claudication, and scalp tenderness.

Consider acute angle-closure glaucoma in painful vision loss with a red eye and nausea.

Summarised Examination

Visual Acuity Test:
- Use a Snellen chart or equivalent to assess vision loss severity.

Pupillary Reflex Testing:
- Look for a relative afferent pupillary defect (RAPD) to identify optic nerve pathology.

Confrontational Visual Field Testing:

Assess for visual field defects (e.g., hemianopia, scotomas).

Ophthalmoscopy:
- Examine retina & optic disc for signs of vascular occlusion, retinal detachment, or swelling.

Peripheral nerve exam

Serious diagnoses to consider

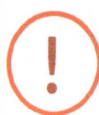

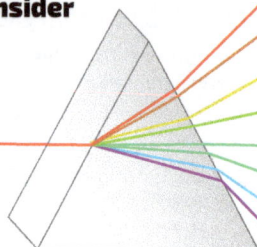

Stroke

Arteritic Anterior Ischaemic Optic Neuropathy (Giant Cell Arteritis)

Retinal Artery Occlusion

Retinal Detachment

Optic Neuritis

Acute Angle-Closure Glaucoma

Retinal Vein Occlusion

Vitreous Haemorrhage

! SERIOUS SYMPTOMS!

Signs and Symptoms

- Painful loss of vision
- Visual field loss after most of vision has returned
- Flashes of light or floaters
- Red eye
- Eye tenderness
- Severe headache
- Jaw pain
- Neurological symptoms

Past medical or surgical history

- Ocular trauma
- Previous eye surgery
- Underlying vascular risk factors: hypertension, diabetes, hyperlipidemia, smoking
- History predisposing them to embolic events: Thrombophilia, Atrial Fibrillation

Diagnostic pathway*

	Symptoms	Examination	Likely Diagnosis
Painful Sudden Loss of Vision	Severe eye pain + headache Nausea and vomiting	 (1) Eye may appear red Fixed and Dilated Corneal oedema	Acute angle-closure glaucoma
	Colour vision impairment (especially red) Painful on eye movement (may be painless)	Potential relative afferent pupillary defect (RAPD) (often hard to see)	Optic neuritis
Painless Sudden Loss of Vision	Temporal headache Jaw claudication	Scalp tenderness Fundoscopy: pale (chalky), swollen optic discs in advanced disease	arteritic anterior ischaemic optic neuropathy (Giant Cell Arteritis)
	Monocular vision loss often described as blurriness Patients typically become aware of this upon waking	decreased visual acuity, dyschromatopsia, an RAPD Fundoscopy: swollen optic nerve with splinter haemorrhages	non-arteritic anterior ischaemic optic neuropathy
	Visual field or monocular vision loss associated with neurological symptoms such as weakness, speech difficulty or dizziness	Neurological exam may reveal signs of stroke (e.g. facial droop, weakness, slurred speech)	Stroke
	Monocular sudden loss of vision	 (2) Fundoscopy - Cherry red spot - Retinal pallor	Retinal Artery Occlusion
	Monocular sudden loss of part of visual field or all of vision, often complaint is blurred vision	 (3) CRVO (4) BRVO Fundoscopy: retinal haemorrhage	Retinal Vein Occlusion

Flashes of light, floaters, and a dark "curtain" descending over part of the visual field	Asymmetrical red reflex Fundoscopy: Detached retinal folds (5)	Retinal Detachment
Blurred vision, sudden appearance of multiple floaters	Darkened or diminished red reflex compared to other eye (6)	Vitreous Haemorrhage

Top tips

- Visual field defects may persist even after partial recovery—always assess thoroughly.
- Always consider Giant Cell Arteritis in patients over 50 with vision loss, as early steroid treatment can prevent blindness.
- Monocular vision loss suggests a lesion anterior to the optic chiasm (e.g., retinal or optic nerve issues).
- Bilateral, symmetrical visual field defects suggest a lesion posterior to the optic chiasm (e.g. occipital lobe stroke).
- Constant eye pain suggests conditions like corneal lesions, anterior chamber inflammation, or acute angle-closure glaucoma.
- Not all optic neuritis presents with pain. Inflammation of the optic nerve can happen at the optic nerve head (papillitis) and/or the optic nerve behind the eye (retrobulbar optic neuritis). Papillitis typically presents with subacute vision loss and a swollen optic disc on fundoscopy. Retrobulbar optic neuritis presents with similar subacute vision loss to papillitis though with the addition of pain on eye movement, optic discs would be normal on fundoscopy.
- Amaurosis fugax refers to a temporary, brief loss of vision in one eye. It is a type of TIA. It is often an early sign of arteritic anterior ischaemic optic neuropathy (AAION) and impending severe vision loss.
- RAPD is an asymmetrical pupillary response to light shone in the eye. This is due to retinal OR optic nerve disease (occurring prior to the lateral geniculate nucleus) that is worse in one eye than the other. All of the conditions listed in the "diagnostic pathway" other than a vitreous haemorrhage will cause a RAPD.
- Examinations for visual defects can be daunting due to length and difficulty of the exam, when short for time ensure to at least do these key steps:
  - Visual acuity
  - Pupillary Reflex testing (RAPD)
  - Confrontational visual fields
  - Peripheral nerve exam
  - If capable: Ophthalmoscopy

Differential diagnoses using the Vitamin C framework

Category	Differential Diagnosis
V - Vascular	Stroke, retinal artery occlusion, retinal vein occlusion, vitreous haemorrhage
I - Infectious	Endophthalmitis, orbital cellulitis
T - Trauma	Vitreous haemorrhage post-trauma
A - Autoimmune	Giant cell arteritis
M - Metabolic	Hyperglycemia-related transient vision loss
I - Idiopathic/Functional	Non-organic vision loss
N - Neoplastic	Optic pathway glioma, metastatic tumors
C - Congenital	Congenital optic nerve anomalies
Other	Retinal detachment, optic neuritis, acute angle-closure glaucoma

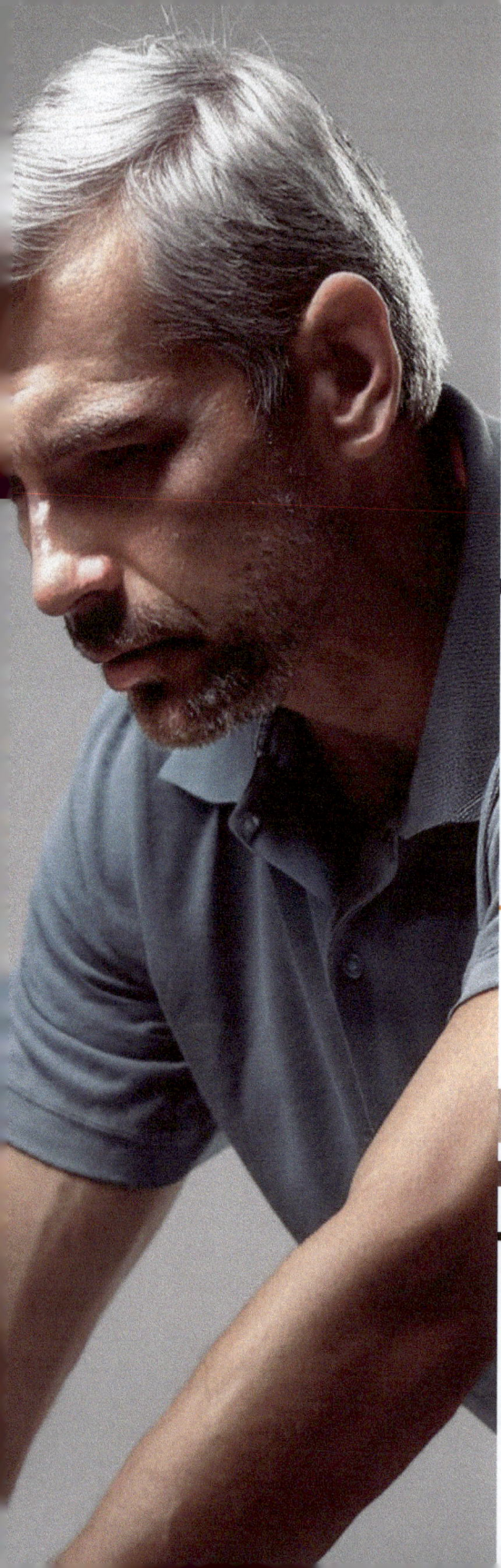

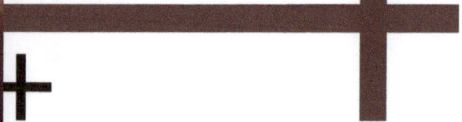

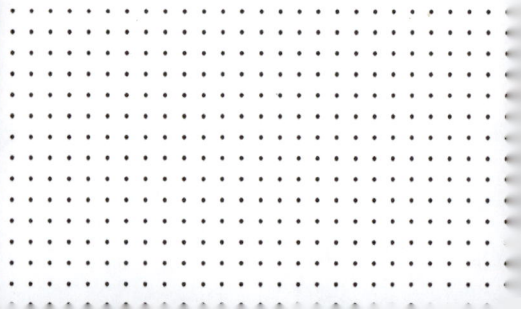

23

Ataxia

Ataxia is a neurological condition characterized by impaired coordination and balance. It arises from dysfunction in the cerebellum, its pathways, or sensory systems, and can result from a wide range of acute, chronic, or progressive conditions. Ataxia may present as isolated unsteadiness, clumsiness, or as part of a broader neurological syndrome. A structured approach to history-taking, examination, and investigation is essential to identify serious causes such as stroke, tumors, or metabolic disorders, and to ensure timely and appropriate management.

Sudden onset

Progressive/worsening Ataxia

Headache

Vomiting

Cranial nerve deficits
e.g. dysphagia, dysarthria, double
vision (diplopia), or weakness

Cerebellar signs -> dysarthria,
nystagmus, dysdiadokinesia, past-
pointing, intention tremor

Ataxia Red Flags

Saddle anaesthesia

Sensory level

Incontinence

Trauma

Systemic illness ->
fever, weight loss

Cancer

Abnormal eye movements
e.g., nystagmus, ophthalmoplegia

Psychiatric Symptoms

History Taking - Important points

- Onset, progression, and duration of ataxia (sudden vs. gradual, progressive vs. intermittent).
- Associated symptoms such as weakness, dysarthria, dysphagia, sensory changes, or other neurological deficits.
- Past medical history including stroke, metabolic diseases, neurological conditions, and substance use (e.g., alcohol or drug use).
- Family history of neurological disorders or inherited ataxias.
- Recent infections, vaccinations, head trauma, or any exposure to toxins or medications.
- Environmental or occupational exposures (e.g., lead, chemicals).
- Any signs of systemic illness like cancer, autoimmune diseases, or liver disease (e.g., Wilson's disease).

Symptoms of serious diagnoses

Rapid onset ataxia, particularly if with other neurological deficits: **Acute stroke, brain haemorrhage, or a space-occupying lesion** (tumour, abscess).

Gradual onset ataxia, progressive worsening: **Neurodegenerative disorders** (spinocerebellar ataxias, multiple system atrophy), **cerebellar degeneration, or chronic metabolic disturbances** (vitamin B12 deficiency).

Ataxia with new, severe unexplained headache & vomiting: **Brain tumour, cerebellar stroke, or increased intracranial pressure**.

Ataxia with cranial nerve deficits (i.e. dysphagia, dysarthria, diplopia) or weakness: **Brainstem stroke, multiple sclerosis, or brainstem tumors**.

Recent head trauma/fall: **Traumatic brain injury, subdural or epidural hematoma, or post-concussion syndrome**.

Ataxia with systemic signs (fever, weight loss) or new-onset weakness: **Infectious causes** (meningitis, encephalitis), **autoimmune disorders** (paraneoplastic syndromes), or **metabolic encephalopathy.**

Cancer with potential for brain metastasis: **Cerebellar metastasis, paraneoplastic syndromes.**

Ataxia in the context of heavy alcohol use or exposure to toxic substances: **Alcohol-related cerebellar degeneration, intoxication, or vitamin deficiencies** (Wernicke's encephalopathy).

Persistent or worsening ataxia despite rest: Acute cerebellar degeneration, progressive neurological conditions, or a space-occupying lesion.

Abnormal eye movements (e.g., nystagmus, ophthalmoplegia): Cerebellar or brainstem lesions, multiple sclerosis, or vestibular disorders.

Ataxia with a **family history of inherited neurological disorders**: Spinocerebellar ataxias, Friedreich's ataxia, or other genetic conditions.

Ataxia in the absence of a clear peripheral cause, such as vertigo, weakness, or sensory loss: Central nervous system lesions, including those affecting the cerebellum or its connections.

Differential diagnoses

I. CENTRAL CAUSES OF ATAXIA

These involve lesions in the brain or spinal cord, particularly affecting the cerebellum, brainstem, or their connections.

CEREBELLAR ATAXIA

Cerebellar Stroke (ischemic or haemor-rhagic)

- Sudden onset, often associated with other neurological deficits (e.g., dysarthria, hemiparesis).
- Imaging: MRI brain is the imaging of

Serious diagnoses to consider

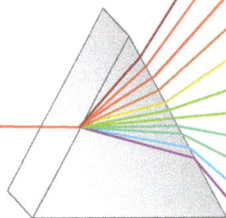

Stroke (Cerebellar or Brainstem Stroke)

Brain Tumour (Primary or Metastatic)

Meningitis/Encephalitis

Acute Cerebellar Ataxia

Wernicke's Encephalopathy (Thiamine Deficiency)

Multiple System Atrophy (MSA)

Guillain-Barré Syndrome (GBS)

Acute Disseminated Encephalomyelitis (ADEM)

Wilson's Disease

Paraneoplastic Cerebellar Degeneration

Infectious Cerebellitis (e.g., Viral Infections)

Differential diagnoses of ataxia

Category	Conditions
V - Vascular	Cerebellar stroke (ischemic or hemorrhagic), Brainstem stroke, Posterior circulation stroke, Cerebral vasculitis
I - Infectious	Meningitis, Encephalitis, Infectious cerebellitis (e.g., Varicella Zoster Virus, Lyme disease), Brain abscess
T - Trauma	Traumatic brain injury (TBI), Subdural or epidural hematoma, Spinal cord trauma
A - Autoimmune	Multiple sclerosis, Acute disseminated encephalomyelitis (ADEM), Paraneoplastic cerebellar degeneration, Guillain-Barré syndrome (GBS), Sarcoidosis
M - Metabolic	Wernicke's encephalopathy (thiamine deficiency), Hypoglycemia, Hypercalcemia, Wilson's disease, Hypothyroidism, Mitochondrial disorders
I - Idiopathic	Functional (psychogenic) ataxia, Sporadic spinocerebellar ataxia, Chronic idiopathic peripheral neuropathy
N - Neoplastic	Brain tumors (primary or metastatic), Paraneoplastic syndromes, Medulloblastoma, Lymphoma, Spinal cord tumors
D - Degenerative	Spinocerebellar ataxias (e.g., SCA1, SCA3), Friedreich's ataxia, Parkinson's disease with cerebellar features, Alcoholic cerebellar degeneration
C - Congenital	Chiari malformation, Arnold-Chiari malformation, Cerebellar hypoplasia, Congenital mitochondrial disorders, Congenital cerebellar malformations

choice.

Cerebellar Degeneration

- Spinocerebellar Ataxias (SCA) (e.g., SCA1, SCA2, SCA3, Friedreich's ataxia)
- Genetic disorders with progressive cerebellar dysfunction, often accompanied by dysarthria, limb ataxia, and sometimes peripheral neuropathy or cardiac issues.
- Diagnosis: Genetic testing and MRI (may show cerebellar atrophy).

Multiple System Atrophy (MSA)

- A progressive neurodegenerative disorder characterized by cerebellar ataxia, parkinsonism, autonomic dysfunction, and sometimes dystonia.
- Diagnosis: MRI shows atrophy of the putamen and cerebellum.

Alcoholic Cerebellar Degeneration

- Chronic alcohol use leads to progressive cerebellar atrophy, particularly in the anterior vermis, resulting in ataxia.
- History of heavy alcohol use and characteristic MRI findings.

Wilson's Disease

- A metabolic disorder with copper accumulation affecting the liver, brain, and corneas, leading to dysarthria, dystonia, and ataxia.
- Diagnosis: Serum ceruloplasmin, urinary copper, liver function tests, and slit-lamp examination (for Kayser-Fleischer rings).

Hypothyroidism

- Severe hypothyroidism can cause cerebellar ataxia due to the direct effects of hypothyroidism on cerebellar function.
- Diagnosis: TSH, T4, T3 levels.

Paraneoplastic Cerebellar Degeneration

- A rare but serious complication of cancer, often associated with antibodies against cerebellar proteins (e.g., anti-Yo, anti-Hu).
- Associated with small cell lung cancer, ovarian cancer, or breast cancer.
- Diagnosis: MRI and serologic testing for paraneoplastic antibodies.

Multiple Sclerosis (MS)

- Can cause ataxia due to demyelination of cerebellar pathways or brainstem.
- Diagnosis: MRI showing multiple white matter lesions, especially in the periventricular region.

BRAINSTEM ATAXIA

Stroke of the Brainstem

- A stroke in the pons or medulla can lead to ataxia along with other deficits (e.g., cranial nerve palsies, weakness).
- Diagnosis: MRI or CT of the brain.

Brainstem Tumours

- Primary brain tumours (e.g., gliomas, brainstem gliomas) or metastases can present with ataxia due to compression of the brainstem.
- Diagnosis: MRI or CT brain

2. PERIPHERAL CAUSES OF ATAXIA

These involve peripheral nerve or vestibular system dysfunction.

VESTIBULAR DISORDERS

Benign Paroxysmal Positional Vertigo (BPPV)

- Episodes of dizziness and unsteadiness triggered by head movements, typically no long-term ataxia.
- Diagnosis: Dix-Hallpike manoeuvre.

Vestibular Neuritis/Labyrinthitis

- Acute onset of vertigo, nausea, and imbalance, usually following a viral infection.
- Diagnosis: Clinical diagnosis; MRI if central pathology is suspected.

Meniere's Disease

- Episodic vertigo associated with tinnitus, hearing loss, and aural fullness.
- Diagnosis: Clinical, often supported by audiometric testing.

Vestibular Schwannoma

- Tumour affecting the vestibulocochlear nerve, leading to vertigo, hearing loss, and imbalance.
- Diagnosis: MRI of the brain with

gadolinium contrast.

PERIPHERAL NEUROPATHY
Chronic Inflammatory Demyelinating Polyneuropathy (CIDP)

- A progressive autoimmune disorder that affects both sensory and motor nerves, leading to ataxia, weakness, and sensory loss.
- Diagnosis: Nerve conduction studies and lumbar puncture showing elevated protein without pleocytosis.

Guillain-Barré Syndrome (GBS)

- A post-infectious autoimmune polyneuropathy that can cause ataxia, weakness, and areflexia.
- Diagnosis: Nerve conduction studies and CSF analysis showing albumin cytologic dissociation.

Charcot-Marie-Tooth Disease (CMT)

- A group of inherited disorders leading to peripheral neuropathy, muscle weakness, and ataxia.
- Diagnosis: Genetic testing, nerve conduction studies, and clinical examination.

Vitamin Deficiencies

- Vitamin B12 deficiency and Vitamin E deficiency can cause ataxia due to sensory and motor neuropathy or spinal cord dysfunction (e.g., subacute combined degeneration in B12 deficiency).
- Diagnosis: Serum B12 and Vitamin E levels, MRI for subacute combined degeneration.

3. SPINAL CORD DISORDERS
Spinal Cord Compression

- Can cause ataxia due to the involvement of the proprioceptive pathways in the dorsal columns.
- Diagnosis: MRI of the spine.

Syringomyelia

- A cyst or cavity forms within the spinal cord, often associated with scoliosis and progressive motor and sensory loss.
- Diagnosis: MRI of the cervical spine.

Multiple Sclerosis (MS)

- MS can also cause spinal cord involvement, resulting in ataxia, weakness, and sensory loss.
- Diagnosis: MRI with gadolinium.

4. METABOLIC AND TOXIC CAUSES
Hypoglycaemia

- Severe hypoglycaemia can cause confusion, ataxia, and other neurological symptoms.
- Diagnosis: Serum glucose levels.

Wernicke's Encephalopathy

- Thiamine deficiency (commonly due to alcohol abuse) can cause ataxia, confusion, and ophthalmoplegia.
- Diagnosis: Clinical diagnosis, response to thiamine supplementation, MRI.

Lead Poisoning

- Chronic exposure to lead can cause ataxia, neuropathy, and cognitive deficits.
- Diagnosis: Blood lead levels.

Mitochondrial Disorders

- Leigh's disease and other mitochondrial disorders can present with progressive ataxia.
- Diagnosis: Genetic testing and mitochondrial enzyme assays.

5. INFECTIOUS CAUSES
Meningitis/Encephalitis

- Can present with ataxia along with fever, headache, and altered mental status.
- Diagnosis: Lumbar puncture and CSF analysis (e.g., PCR, cultures).

Varicella Zoster Virus (VZV)

- VZV infection can cause cerebellar ataxia, especially in immunocompromised patients.
- Diagnosis: PCR or serology for VZV.

Lyme Disease

- Can cause ataxia as part of Lyme neuroborreliosis.
- Diagnosis: Serology for Lyme disease, PCR, or CSF analysis.

6. PSYCHIATRIC CAUSES

Functional (Psychogenic) Ataxia

- Patients may have apparent ataxia with no clear neurological cause, often exacerbated by stress.
- Diagnosis: Exclusion of organic causes through detailed neurological evaluation and observation.

KEY INVESTIGATIONS

- MRI Brain (preferred for central causes)
- CT Brain (if acute stroke or haemorrhage is suspected)
- Lumbar Puncture (if an infectious or inflammatory cause is suspected)
- Blood Tests (including B12, thyroid function, electrolytes, liver function, etc.)
- Genetic Testing (if hereditary ataxia is suspected)
- Nerve Conduction Studies (if peripheral neuropathy is suspected)

SENSORY ATAXIA

- Patterns of sensory deficit causing sensory ataxia: Glove and stocking in peripheral neuropathy ,hemi sensory loss in cortical lesion and sensory level with para sensory loss in spinal cord lesions.
- For normal movement, proprioception and cerebellum has to work in conjunction with inputs to and fro from the brain. In the presence of profound sensory loss particularly in he hands and feet, interferes with fine motor skills in he hands, and with Standing and walking when involving the feet.
- The patient compensates by using his eyes to monitor movement of the hands or feet. As a result the clumsiness or unsteadiness gets worse in he dark or at times when eyes are closed e.g while having a bath.

Glove and stocking in peripheral neuropathy

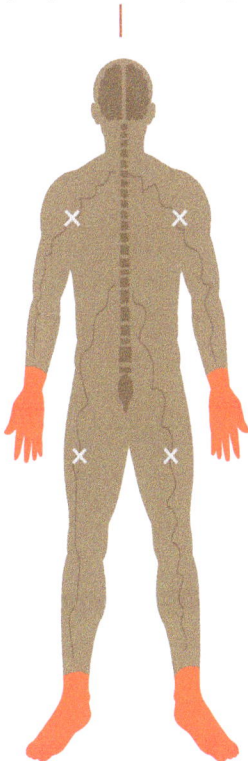

Para sensory loss in spinal cord lesions.

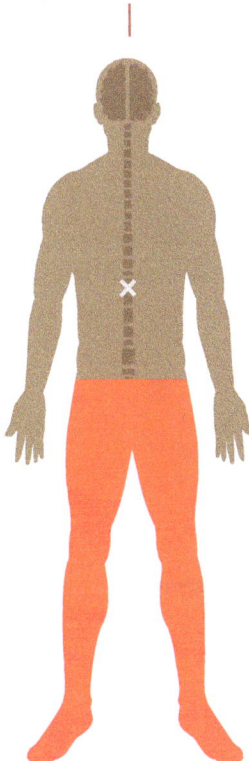

Hemi sensory loss in cortical lesion

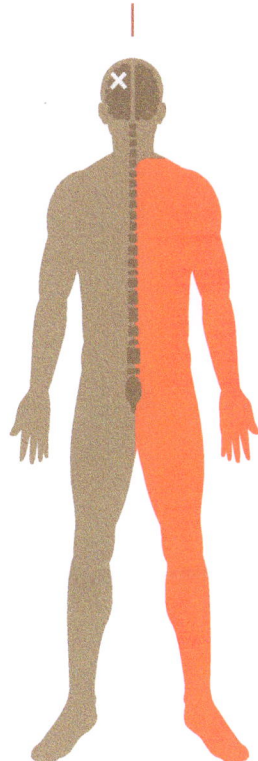

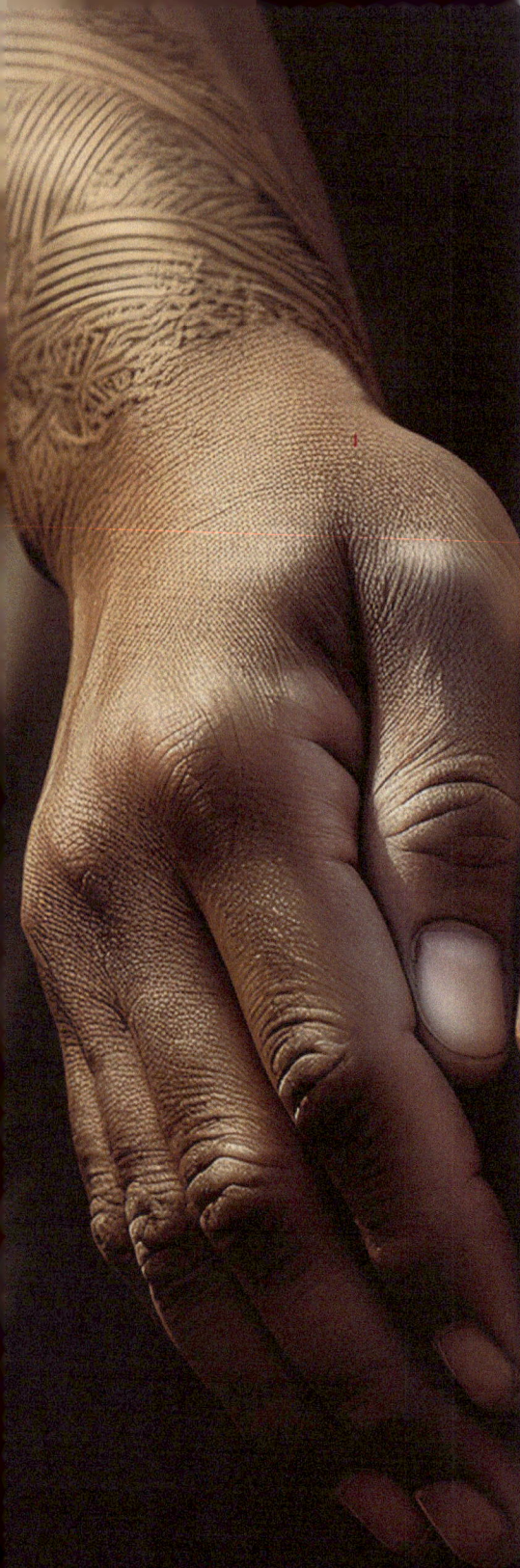

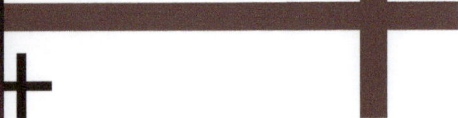

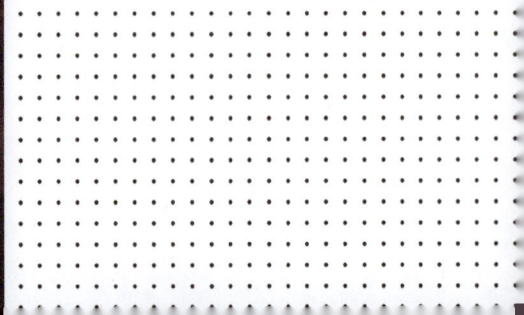

24

Tremor

Tremor is an involuntary, rhythmic movement of a body part, often presenting as a standalone symptom or as part of a broader neurological, systemic, or metabolic condition. While most tremors, such as essential tremor, are benign, others may indicate serious underlying disorders like Parkinson's disease, stroke, or systemic illnesses. Early identification of red flags and a detailed assessment of the tremor type—resting, postural, or action—can guide timely and appropriate investigations, improving patient outcomes.

Tremor Red Flags

- Sudden onset

- Neurological Deficits -> muscle weakness, dysarthria, ataxia, vision changes, or balance issues

- Cognitive or Personality Changes

- Under 40

- Bradykinesia or Rigidity

- Changes in Gait or Posture

- Weight Loss

- Night Sweats

- Fever

- Hallucinations

- Autonomic Dysfunction -> dizziness, fainting, constipation, or urinary incontinence

History Taking - Important points

ONSET AND TIMING:

- Is the tremor acute or gradual? Did it start suddenly or slowly progress over time?

TYPE OF TREMOR:

- Is it resting, action, or postural? Does it worsen with certain movements (intention tremor)?

ASSOCIATED FEATURES:

- Are there additional neurological signs (e.g., weakness, gait changes, cognitive decline), systemic symptoms (e.g., weight loss, sweating), or any changes in mood, cognition, or behaviour?
- Does alcohol improve the Tremor? Essential Tremor
- which body part are affected? The

Laryngeal muscles and tongue may be involved in essential tremor causing a tremor in voice . A head tremor is also associated with essential tremor.

MEDICATION HISTORY:

- Any recent drug use or withdrawal? History of alcohol or substance abuse?

FAMILY HISTORY:

- Is there a family history of movement disorders or neurological conditions?

AGE AND RISK FACTORS:

- Consider the patient's age, occupation, and any potential history of head trauma or occupational exposure.

Symptoms suggestive of serious diagnoses

- Sudden, particularly if it's isolated to one side of the body or associated with other neurological signs (e.g., weakness, speech difficulties): may indicate a **stroke or acute neurological event, such as a brain haemorrhage or acute parkinsonism.**
- Associated with Neurological Deficits (e.g., muscle weakness, speech difficulties, vision changes, or balance issues): This could suggest **multiple sclerosis, stroke, brain tumor, or neurodegenerative diseases like Parkinson's disease or progressive supranuclear palsy.**
- Accompanied by cognitive decline, confusion, memory problems, or personality changes: These may point to **neurodegenerative conditions** such as **Parkinson's disease with dementia, Lewy body dementia, or Alzheimer's disease.**
- Tremor occurring in a young patient (especially under age 40) without a family history of tremors or neurodegenerative disease: Could suggest genetic disorders like **Wilson's disease (copper buildup), early-onset Parkinson's disease, or dystonia.** It may also indicate **essential tremor or drug-induced tremor.**
- A resting tremor (e.g., pill-rolling tremor) that is associated with bradykinesia (slowness of movement), rigidity, or postural instability: These are hallmark features of **Parkinson's disease or other parkinsonian syndromes,** which require specific management and monitoring.
- Development of a tremor in the presence of gait abnormalities, postural instability, or difficulty with coordination: This could indicate **Parkinson's disease, cerebellar disorders, or degenerative conditions like multiple system atrophy (MSA).**
- If tremor is accompanied by significant weight loss, night sweats, or unexplained fever, this suggests an infectious or systemic cause: **Hyperthyroidism or thyrotoxicosis can cause tremors. Additionally, malignancy (e.g., paraneoplastic syndrome) or infectious encephalitis** might present with tremor.
- Tremor combined with hallucinations or delusions: Could be a feature of **Parkinson's disease with psychosis, Lewy body dementia, or drug-induced tremors** from antipsychotics or other medications.
- A tremor that doesn't respond to common

Serious diagnoses to consider

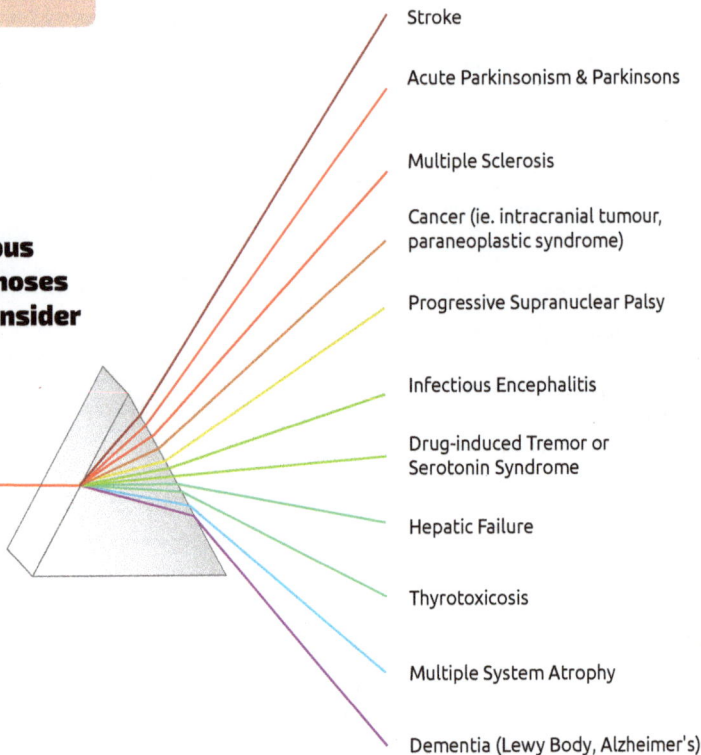

Stroke

Acute Parkinsonism & Parkinsons

Multiple Sclerosis

Cancer (ie. intracranial tumour, paraneoplastic syndrome)

Progressive Supranuclear Palsy

Infectious Encephalitis

Drug-induced Tremor or Serotonin Syndrome

Hepatic Failure

Thyrotoxicosis

Multiple System Atrophy

Dementia (Lewy Body, Alzheimer's)

Differential diagnoses of tremor

Category	Conditions
V - Vascular	Stroke (cerebellar or basal ganglia), Arteriovenous malformations (AVM)
I - Infectious	Infectious encephalitis (e.g., Japanese encephalitis), Paraneoplastic syndromes with infectious features
T - Trauma	Post-traumatic tremor, Chronic traumatic encephalopathy (CTE)
A - Autoimmune	Multiple sclerosis, Paraneoplastic syndromes, Systemic lupus erythematosus (SLE)
M - Metabolic	Thyrotoxicosis, Wilson's disease, Hypoglycemia, Hyperadrenergic states (e.g., pheochromocytoma, panic attacks)
I - Idiopathic	Essential tremor, Functional (psychogenic) tremor
N - Neoplastic	Brain tumors (e.g., gliomas, metastatic lesions), Paraneoplastic syndromes
D - Degenerative	Parkinson's disease, Multiple system atrophy (MSA), Progressive supranuclear palsy (PSP), Huntington's disease
C - Congenital	Dystonia-parkinsonism syndromes, Hereditary spinocerebellar ataxias

treatments, especially in the case of medications that should generally reduce tremor: This may indicate a more severe or atypical form of a tremor disorder, such as **tremor-dominant Parkinson's disease, progressive supranuclear palsy, or multiple system atrophy (MSA)**.

- A strong family history of tremors or movement disorders (especially in the absence of other signs): A family history of essential tremor, Parkinson's disease, or other hereditary tremor syndromes can point to a genetic cause that may require specialized testing or management.
- Tremor accompanied by autonomic symptoms such as dizziness, fainting, constipation, or urinary incontinence: This could point to **multiple system atrophy (MSA) or Parkinson's disease**, as these conditions can impact both the nervous system and autonomic functions.
- Tremor that is associated with certain activities, particularly if it worsens with postural changes (e.g., holding a position, performing fine motor tasks): This may be characteristic of **essential tremor or task-specific tremor**, and requires differentiation from more serious conditions like **cerebellar ataxia or neurodegenerative diseases**.
- Recent onset of tremor in patients who have started new medications, especially those with dopaminergic effects (e.g., antipsychotics, antiemetics), or illicit drug use (e.g., methamphetamine): This could be indicative of **drug-induced tremor or serotonin syndrome**.

Differential diagnoses

I. NEURODEGENERATIVE DISORDERS
Parkinson's Disease (PD)

- Tremor Type: Resting tremor (e.g., pill-rolling tremor).
- Other Features: Bradykinesia, rigidity, postural instability, and micrographia. Symmetric tremor with asymmetry of motor signs often seen in early stages.

Essential Tremor (ET)

- Tremor Type: Postural and action tremor, usually affecting the hands, head, or voice.
- Other Features: Worsens with movement and improves at rest, often familial.

Multiple System Atrophy (MSA)

- Tremor Type: Resting or postural tremor.
- Other Features: Autonomic dysfunction (e.g., orthostatic hypotension), cerebellar ataxia, and parkinsonism.

Progressive Supranuclear Palsy (PSP)

- Tremor Type: Less common, but may be present as postural tremor.
- Other Features: Vertical gaze palsy, postural instability, axial rigidity, early falls, and cognitive decline.

Corticobasal Degeneration (CBD)

- Tremor Type: May include asymmetric action tremor or dystonic tremor.
- Other Features: Limb apraxia, dystonia, asymmetric rigidity, alien limb phenomenon, and cognitive changes.

2. CEREBELLAR DISORDERS
Cerebellar Ataxia (e.g., spinocerebellar ataxia, cerebellar degeneration)

- Tremor Type: Intention tremor (worsens with voluntary movement).
- Other Features: Ataxia, dysmetria (inability to judge distances), dysarthria, and imbalance.

Multiple Sclerosis (MS)

- Tremor Type: Intention tremor.
- Other Features: History of relapsing-remitting neurological symptoms (e.g., optic neuritis, weakness, numbness), and cerebellar signs.

3. METABOLIC/ENDOCRINE DISORDERS
Thyrotoxicosis (Hyperthyroidism)

- Tremor Type: Fine resting or postural tremor.

- Other Features: Weight loss, heat intolerance, tachycardia, palpitations, and increased sweating.

Wilson's Disease

- Tremor Type: Action or postural tremor, often asymmetrical.
- Other Features: Hepatic dysfunction (cirrhosis, jaundice), neuropsychiatric symptoms (mood changes, personality changes), and dystonia.

Hypoglycemia

- Tremor Type: Fine tremor, often with hypoglycemic symptoms (e.g., sweating, confusion, tachycardia).
- Other Features: History of diabetes or insulin use, fasting, or excessive alcohol consumption.

4. TOXIC AND DRUG-INDUCED TREMORS

Medications

- Tremor Type: Can be rest, postural, or action tremor depending on the drug.
- Other Features: Associated with specific drugs, including dopamine antagonists (e.g., antipsychotics like haloperidol, metoclopramide), SSRIs, lithium, stimulants (e.g., caffeine, amphetamines), and anticonvulsants.

Withdrawal Syndromes

- Tremor Type: Fine tremor, often seen with alcohol or benzodiazepine withdrawal.
- Other Features: Anxiety, agitation, tachycardia, and autonomic instability.

Heavy Metal Poisoning (e.g., lead, mercury)

- Tremor Type: Action or postural tremor.
- Other Features: Neurological signs such as peripheral neuropathy, gait disturbance, and cognitive decline.

5. VASCULAR DISORDERS

Stroke (Ischemic or Hemorrhagic)

- Tremor Type: Often postural or intentional tremor if the cerebellum or basal ganglia is affected.
- Other Features: Sudden onset of focal neurological signs, such as weakness, sensory changes, dysphasia, or visual changes.

Arteriovenous Malformations (AVM)

- Tremor Type: Action or postural tremor, depending on location.
- Other Features: Seizures, headache, or focal neurological deficits, often with a history of previous haemorrhage.

6. SYSTEMIC AND INFECTIOUS CAUSES

Paraneoplastic Syndromes

- Tremor Type: Can vary, often postural or action tremor.
- Other Features: Weight loss, fatigue, and other systemic signs of malignancy (e.g., lung, breast, or ovarian cancer).

Infectious Encephalitis

- Tremor Type: Can be part of the spectrum of movement disorders seen in encephalitis (e.g., Japanese encephalitis).
- Other Features: Fever, altered mental status, focal neurological deficits, and seizures.

7. PSYCHOGENIC TREMOR (FUNCTIONAL TREMOR)

- Tremor Type: Can be rest, postural, or action tremor, often variable or inconsistent.
- Other Features: Tremor may improve with distraction or suggestibility. Often associated with psychological stress or trauma. May be part of a functional movement disorder (FMD).

8. TRAUMA OR INJURY

Post-Traumatic Tremor

- Tremor Type: Can be action or postural tremor.
- Other Features: A history of head injury or repetitive head trauma (e.g., from boxing or football).

Chronic Traumatic Encephalopathy (CTE)

- Tremor Type: May include tremor as part of a broader constellation of movement and cognitive symptoms.
- Other Features: Cognitive decline, mood

changes, and a history of repetitive head trauma.

9. PERIPHERAL NERVOUS SYSTEM DISORDERS

Peripheral Neuropathy

- Tremor Type: May include action tremor, but more often associated with other signs like weakness or numbness.
- Other Features: Sensory loss, loss of reflexes, and other signs of peripheral nerve involvement.

10. GENETIC DISORDERS

Dystonia-Parkinsonism Syndromes (e.g., Wilson's Disease, Huntington's Disease)

- Tremor Type: Can be action or postural tremor, often with dystonia.
- Other Features: Family history, other movement abnormalities (e.g., chorea, dystonia), and progressive nature of the disorder.

11. MISCELLANEOUS CAUSES

Functional Tremor (Psychogenic Tremor)

- Tremor Type: Inconsistent tremor that may change with distraction.
- Other Features: Often occurs in the context of psychological stress or trauma. History may be inconsistent or highly suggestive of psychological causes.

Fibromyalgia

- Tremor Type: Sometimes seen as a generalized fine tremor.
- Other Features: Widespread pain, sleep disturbances, and fatigue.

12. HYPERADRENERGIC STATES

Panic Attacks

- Tremor Type: Fine, resting tremor, often associated with anxiety.
- Other Features: Palpitations, shortness of breath, chest tightness, and acute onset of anxiety.

Pheochromocytoma

- Tremor Type: Fine tremor, often associated with other adrenergic symptoms.
- Other Features: Episodic hypertension, palpitations, sweating, and headaches.

Top tips

The presence of any of these red flags—particularly if they suggest a more serious neurological, systemic, or degenerative cause—requires prompt and thorough investigation. If a tremor is accompanied by sudden neurological changes, significant cognitive issues, or autonomic dysfunction, early referral to a neurologist is crucial for further workup and management.

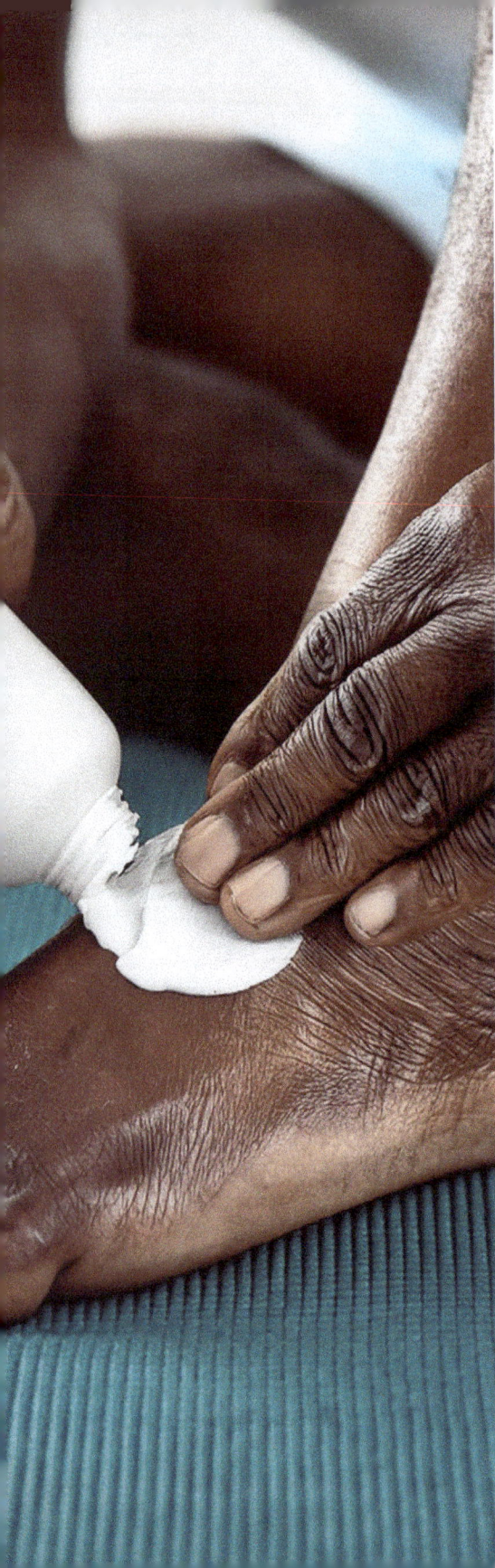

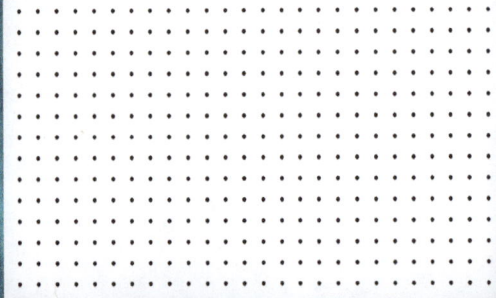

25

Numbness and paraesthesia

Numbness and paraesthesia are common neurological complaints that range from benign and transient to indicators of serious underlying pathology. These symptoms, characterized by altered sensation such as tingling or a "pins and needles" feeling, can result from peripheral nerve damage, central nervous system disorders, or systemic conditions. A structured history and examination, along with attention to red flags, are essential to distinguish between benign and critical causes, ensuring timely diagnosis and treatment.

Diagnostic sieves

Paraesthesia Red Flags

Central Neurological Symptoms

- Sudden onset numbness or paraesthesia
- Weakness affecting one side of the body
- Facial weakness
- Confusion or loss of consciousness
- Slurred speech
- Vision loss or changes

Spinal Neurological Symptoms

- Saddle anaesthesia
- Loss of bladder or bowel control
- Numbness following recent head, neck, or back trauma

Motor and Mobility Issues

- Difficulty walking or limb weakness
- Progressive motor or sensory deficits

Serious diagnoses to consider

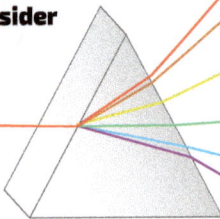

- Multiple Sclerosis
- Spinal Cord Compression (e.g. Cauda Equina Syndrome)
- Guillain-Barré Syndrome
- Brain Tumors
- Nerve Injury (e.g., radial, ulnar, or sciatic nerve)
- Stroke or TIA

History Taking - Important points

1. ONSET AND DURATION
When did the symptoms start?
Was the onset sudden or gradual?
Is it constant, intermittent, or progressive?

2. LOCATION AND DISTRIBUTION
Where exactly is the numbness/paraesthesia?
Is it unilateral or bilateral?
Is it localised (e.g. specific limb or area) or generalised?

3. ASSOCIATED SYMPTOMS
Weakness, clumsiness, or difficulty with movement?
Pain, tingling, or burning sensation?
Loss of bladder or bowel control?
Dizziness, vision changes, or speech difficulty?
Fever, recent infection, or rash?

Fatigue, joint pain, or weight loss?

4. TRIGGERS AND ALLEVIATING FACTORS
Does anything make the symptoms better or worse (e.g. position, activity)?
Any recent injury or trauma?

5. MEDICAL HISTORY
Do you have diabetes, hypertension, or any other chronic illnesses?
Have you had any recent infections or vaccinations?
Have you experienced similar symptoms in the past?

6. MEDICATIONS AND SUBSTANCES
Do you consume alcohol or recreational drugs?

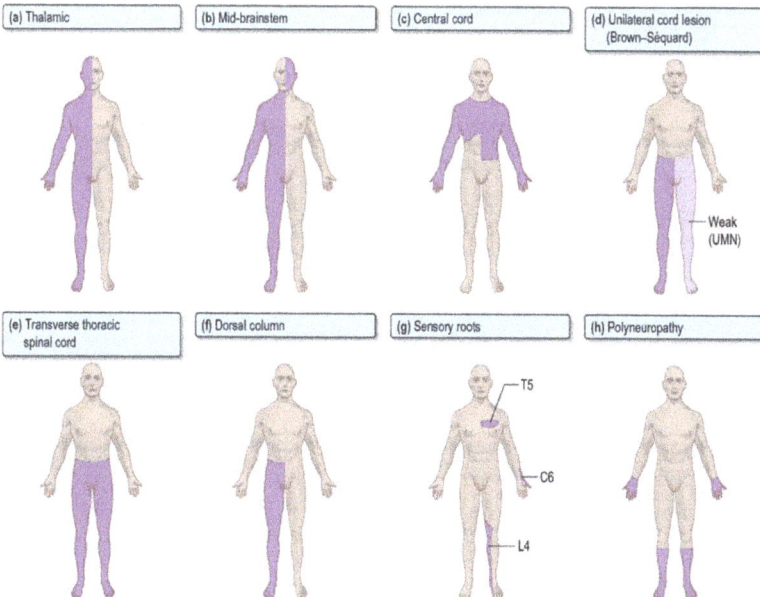

Principal patterns of loss of sensation. (a) **Thalamic lesion:** sensory loss throughout opposite side (rare). (b) **Brainstem lesion:** contralateral sensory loss below face and ipsilateral loss on face. (c) **Central cord lesion,** e.g. syrinx: 'suspended' areas of loss, often asymmetrical and 'dissociated', i.e. pain and temperature loss but light touch intact. (d) **Hemisection of cord/unilateral cord lesion** = Brown–Séquard syndrome: contralateral spinothalamic (pain and temperature) loss with ipsilateral weakness and dorsal column loss below lesion. (e) **Transverse cord lesion:** loss of all modalities, including motor, below lesion. (f) **Dorsal column lesion,** e.g. MS: loss of proprioception, vibration and light touch. (g) **Individual sensory root lesions,** e.g. C6, T5, L4. (h) **Polyneuropathy:** distal sensory loss.

https://www.grepmed.com/images/3568/sensation-distribution-deficit-sensory-neurology

Key differentials

Cause	Key features	Findings	Associated Symptoms	Investigations
Stroke or Transient Ischaemic Attack (TIA)	Sudden onset; hemibody numbness; may include facial droop, slurred speech, or weakness.	Asymmetric motor weakness, cranial nerve deficits.	Confusion, vision changes, dizziness.	CT head (urgent for stroke), MRI brain (preferred if available). ECG: To assess for atrial fibrillation or other arrhythmias.
Multiple sclerosis	Episodic or progressive numbness, often involves multiple body region	Hyperreflexia, Lhermitte's sign (electric shock sensation), visual disturbances	Fatigue, muscle spasms, and bladder dysfunction.	**MRI Brain and Spine**: T2 hyperintense lesions characteristic of MS. **Lumbar Puncture**: Oligoclonal bands in cerebrospinal fluid (CSF).
Peripheral Neuropathy	"Stocking-glove" distribution of numbness; sensory loss is symmetrical.	Diminished vibration sense, reduced/absent reflexes	Burning or tingling pain; may be related to diabetes, alcoholism, or toxins.	**Nerve Conduction Studies (NCS)**: To confirm peripheral neuropathy and determine type (axonal vs. demyelinating). **Blood Tests**: HbA1c, B12, folate, thyroid function tests, and autoimmune panel.
Guillain-Barré Syndrome (GBS)	Rapidly ascending numbness or weakness, often post-infection	Reduced or absent reflexes, symmetric weakness	Difficulty breathing (severe cases)	**Lumbar Puncture**: Elevated CSF protein with normal white cell count. **Blood Tests**: Screen for infections
Cauda Equina Syndrome	Saddle anaesthesia, bowel or bladder dysfunction	Reduced anal tone, bilateral lower limb weakness.	Lower back pain, sciatica	**MRI Spine**: Urgent to assess for compression of cauda equina nerves.
Cervical or Lumbar Radiculopathy	Dermatomal distribution of numbness; may include radicular pain.	Positive Spurling's test, reduced reflexes in affected myotomes.	Pain, weakness in specific nerve root distribution	**MRI Spine**: To identify nerve root compression, disc herniation, or foraminal stenosis.
Transverse Myelitis	Bilateral numbness below a spinal level; may progress rapidly	Sensory level on examination, brisk reflexes below the lesion	Back pain, urinary retention	**MRI Spine**: To detect inflammation in the spinal cord. **Lumbar Puncture**: Raised white cell count or proteins, assess for infectious or autoimmune causes. **Autoimmune Panel**: ANA, anti-dsDNA, NMO-IgG, and myelin oligodendrocyte glycoprotein antibodies.
Vitamin B12 Deficiency	Gradual onset; often with gait instability. Often associated with demographics who are likely to have nutrition deficiencies such as alcoholics	Reduced vibration and position sense, megaloblastic anaemia	Glossitis, fatigue, neuropsychiatric symptoms	Serum B12 levels

Infectious Neuropathies (e.g. Lyme Disease, HIV, Syphilis)	Progressive, focal or diffuse numbness	Rash (Lyme), cranial nerve involvement, lymphadenopathy.	Fever, fatigue, joint pain (Lyme).	**Lyme Disease**: Lyme serology (ELISA, confirm with Western blot). **HIV**: HIV serology. **Syphilis**: Treponemal tests (e.g., TPPA, RPR). **CSF Analysis**: If neurosyphilis or HIV-related neuropathy is suspected.
Spinal Epidural Abscess	Rapid progression; associated back pain	Tender spine, fever, possible sensory level	Fever, localised tenderness	MRI Spine with Contrast **Blood Tests**: CRP, ESR, blood cultures.
Spinal Trauma	Numbness below the level of injury; history of trauma	Neurological deficits, step-off deformities	Paralysis, pain	CT trauma scan, MRI scan to give further insight into cord involvement
Nerve Compression Syndromes (e.g. Carpal Tunnel Syndrome)	Localised numbness; median nerve distribution	Positive Tinel's and Phalen's tests	Pain, tingling in affected area	Nerve conduction studies, ultrasound of the median nerve.
Thoracic Outlet Syndrome	Numbness in the upper limb; positional exacerbation	Diminished pulse with specific manoeuvres	Upper extremity swelling, pain	Duplex ultrasound, MRI/CT angiography if vascular involvement is suspected.
Toxic Neuropathies	Progressive numbness; history of toxin exposure (e.g., heavy metals, chemotherapy)	Diffuse or patchy deficits	Weakness, ataxia	Heavy metal levels (e.g., lead, arsenic), drug levels (e.g., chemotherapy agents).
Functional disorder	Symptoms not consistent with anatomical or physiological patterns	Inconsistent findings on repeat examination	Anxiety, depression or additional serious mental health conditions	Psychiatry referral

Examination

1. **GENERAL OBSERVATIONS**

2. **NEUROLOGICAL EXAMINATION**

- Cranial Nerves: Assess for facial numbness, asymmetry, or eye movement abnormalities (e.g. stroke, multiple sclerosis).
- Motor Function: Test muscle strength in affected and unaffected areas.
- Reflexes: Test deep tendon reflexes (e.g. hyperreflexia in upper motor neuron lesions, dampened reflexes in peripheral neuropathy).
- Sensation: Assess light touch, pinprick, vibration, and proprioception.
- Coordination: Perform finger-to-nose and heel-to-shin tests.
- Gait: Observe walking for unsteadiness or foot drop.

3. SPINE EXAMINATION

- Palpate and inspect for tenderness, deformity, or swelling.
- Assess for signs of spinal cord compression or radiculopathy (e.g. straight leg raise for lumbar nerve root compression).

4. SYSTEMIC EXAMINATION

- Infection Signs: Check for fever, lymphadenopathy, or systemic rash.

- Endocrine/Metabolic Signs: Inspect for signs of hypothyroidism (dry skin, bradycardia) or vitamin B12 deficiency (glossitis).

5. FUNCTIONAL ASSESSMENT

- Evaluate for non-anatomical patterns of numbness or inconsistencies, suggesting a functional neurological disorder.

Top tips

CONSIDER ACUTE VS. CHRONIC:

- Rapid progression over hours to days could indicate serious conditions like Guillain-Barré syndrome, spinal cord compression, or stroke and requires urgent investigation.
- Chronic symptoms may be related to diabetes, nutritional deficiencies, or toxic exposures.

CONSIDERATIONS FOR INVESTIGATIONS:

- Start with basic blood tests (e.g., glucose, vitamin B12, thyroid function)
- Use imaging (MRI or CT) for suspected spinal cord or brain lesions, or nerve compression syndromes.
- Consider lumbar puncture if infection or inflammatory neuropathy (e.g., Guillain-Barré) is suspected.

KNOW WHEN TO REFER:

- Refer urgently for acute, rapidly progressing, or atypical symptoms.
- Consider specialist referral for unclear diagnoses after initial workup, or for management of complex neuropathies.

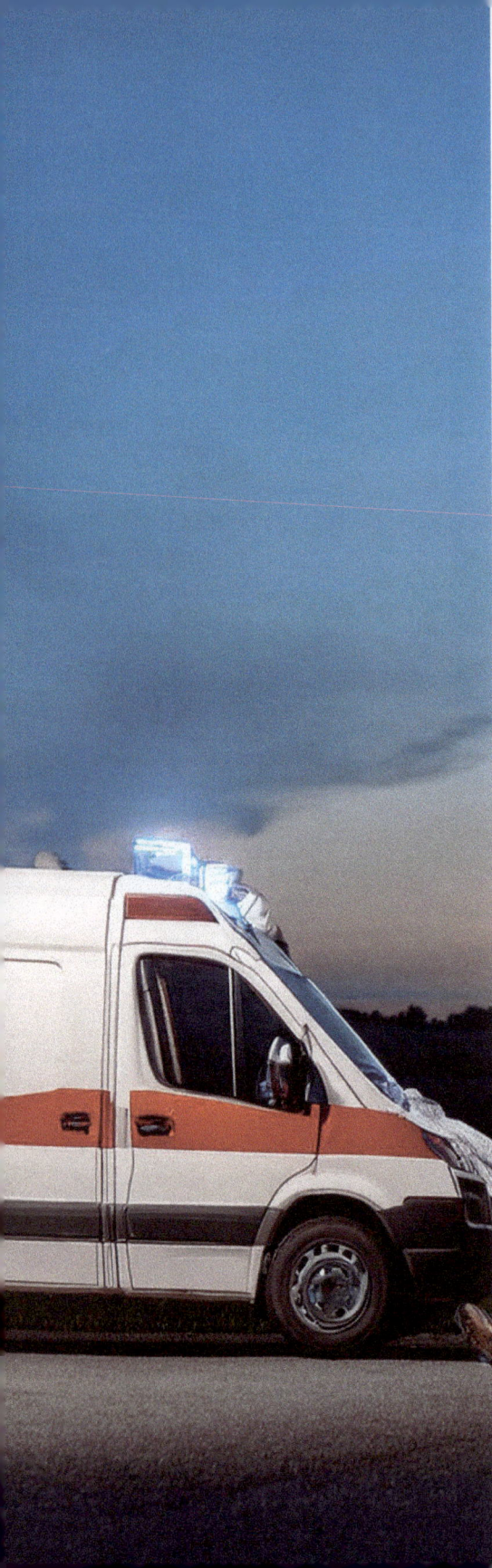

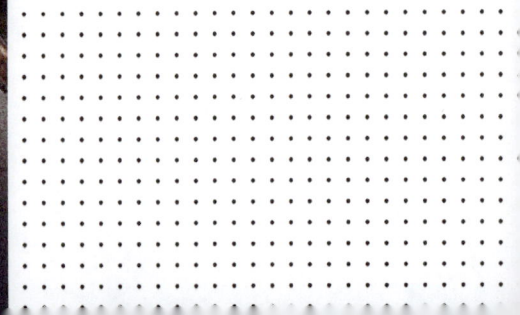

26
Seizure

A **seizure** is an abnormal and excessive electrical discharge in the brain that disrupts normal neuronal activity. Seizures can present as isolated events or as part of an underlying condition like epilepsy, metabolic derangements, or systemic illnesses. Identifying the cause and distinguishing between focal and generalized seizures is crucial for management. Attention to red flags, history, and examination helps prioritize serious conditions such as stroke, infection, or structural brain lesions that may mimic or precipitate seizures.

Diagnostic sieves

Seizure Red Flags

History

- Recent Trauma
- Signs such as fever, neck stiffness, altered mental state, irritability, or a petechial rash
- Seizure activity lasting more than 5 minutes or 3 or more seizures within an hour
- Recurrent seizures
- Seizures without a full recovery
- Associated with chest pain, arrhythmia, or collapse during exercise.
- New seizures in pregnancy or postpartum
- History of malignancy
- Alcohol excess
- Immune suppression
- Associated severe headache

Examination

- GCS Persistently <15
- Focal Neurological Deficit: Persistent weakness, vision changes, or speech problems lasting longer than an hour post-seizure.
- Arrhythmia

History Taking - Important points

1. DETAILS OF THE EVENT

Before
- What was the patient doing before the event?
- Was there any warning (aura, lightheadedness, strange sensations)?
- How long did the episode last?
- Any preceding headache or visual changes?

During
- What did the event look like?
- Was there jerking, rigidity, or loss of consciousness?
- Was there tongue biting, incontinence, or cyanosis?

After
- What was the recovery like, were they fatigued or confused?

2. MEDICAL HISTORY
- Any past episodes? If so, were they similar or different to this one?
- History of stroke, traumatic brain injury, meningitis, or encephalitis.
- Any history of arrhythmias, syncope, or structural heart disease?
- Recent fever, rash, or feeling generally unwell?

3. TRIGGERS OR PROVOKING FACTORS
- Recent sleep deprivation or significant emotional stress?
- Recent alcohol binge or withdrawal? Use of recreational drugs?
- Current medications (e.g., antipsychotics, antibiotics) and adherence to anti-seizure drugs.

4. FAMILY AND SOCIAL HISTORY
- Any family history of epilepsy, sudden unexplained deaths, or cardiac conditions?

5. PREGNANCY-SPECIFIC HISTORY
- How many weeks are you through your pregnancy? Have you ever previously been pregnant? If so, did you have any issues during that pregnancy?

Immediate Seizure Management

EXPOSURE ASSESSMENT AND MANAGE-MENT

Assessment:
- Look for signs of rashes (e.g. meningococcal sepsis)
- Looks for signs of trauma (e.g. fractures, bruising, head injuries)
- Assess temperature (pyrexia may indicate infection or febrile convulsions).

Baseline immediate bloods:
- Full Blood Count + CRP
- Urea & Electrolytes, including Calcium and Magnesium
- Liver Function Tests.
- Blood gas (preferably arterial)- evaluate metabolic or respiratory disturbances

Post Seizure examination
- Monitor the patients observations: ideally cardiac monitoring
- Assess for injury- inspect inside the mouth for lateral tongue bites, look for any trauma to the skin, head or joints
- Assess mental state: Use GCS to assess consciousness and cognitive function
- Auscultate the chest for aspiration- if suspected will require a Chest X-ray
- Cardiac exam: check for signs of arrhythmia or abnormalities- get a 12 lead ECG
- Neurology exam: Perform a neurological exam to identify any focal deficits (e.g. weakness, sensory loss, speech difficulties)

Additional investigations:
- CT/MRI brain (suspected structural pathology).
- EEG (electrical activity abnormalities).
- Lumbar puncture (if CNS infection suspected).

**Serious
diagnoses
to consider**

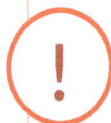

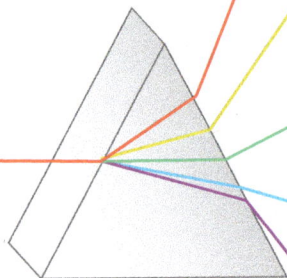

STRUCTURAL CAUSES
- Brain Tumor
- Stroke
- Traumatic Brain Injury
- Intracranial Hemorrhage (Subarachnoid, Subdural, Epidural, or Intracerebral)
- Cerebral Abscess

GENETIC CAUSES
- Epilepsy Syndromes (e.g., Dravet Syndrome, Lennox-Gastaut Syndrome)
- Neurocutaneous Syndromes (e.g., Tuberous Sclerosis, Neurofibromatosis)

INFECTIOUS CAUSES
- Meningitis
- Encephalitis (e.g., viral, bacterial, fungal)
- Cerebral Abscess

IMMUNE CAUSES
- Autoimmune Encephalitis (e.g., anti-NMDA Receptor Encephalitis, Limbic Encephalitis)

HYPOGLYCEMIA OR HYPERG-LYCEMIA
- Electrolyte Imbalances:
    - Hyponatremia, Hypernatremia, Hypocalcemia, Hypercalcemia, Hypomagnesemia
- Uremic Encephalopathy
- Hepatic Encephalopathy
- Eclampsia
- Alcohol Withdrawal
- Drug Overdose or Recreational Drug Use (e.g., cocaine, amphetamines)
- Hypertensive Encephalopathy

Key differentials

Producing the diagnostic algorithm

	Cause	Key features	Findings	Associated Symptoms	Investigations
Neurological Causes	Epilepsy	Unprovoked, recurrent seizures; may be generalized or focal. Aura or postictal state common	Often no additional cause for seizure found	Focal neurological symptoms or developmental delay in some cases	EEG (abnormal interictal activity in epilepsy). MRI brain (to exclude structural lesions)
	Stroke or Transient Ischemic Attack (TIA)	Sudden-onset neurological deficit with focal features	Hemiparesis, facial droop, or aphasia; seizures may follow ischemic changes	Risk factors such as hypertension, atrial fibrillation	CT/MRI brain (acute infarct or haemorrhage)
	Traumatic Brain Injury (TBI)/Intracranial haemorrhage	History of head trauma; may have delayed onset seizures	Signs of head injury, scalp hematoma, or skull fracture	Headache, vomiting, loss of consciousness	CT head (to rule out intracranial haemorrhage)
	Subarachnoid Haemorrhage (SAH)	Sudden "thunderclap" headache; seizures may occur with initial bleed	Neck stiffness, photophobia, decreased consciousness	Nausea, vomiting	CT head (blood in the subarachnoid space) Lumbar puncture (xanthochromia if CT is negative)
	CNS Infections (Meningitis, Encephalitis, Brain Abscess)	Fever, altered mental status, headache; seizures are common in encephalitis and abscess	Neck stiffness (meningitis), focal deficits, or papilledema	Petechial rash (meningitis) Behavioural changes (encephalitis) Confusion or reduced consciousness	Lumbar puncture (CSF analysis) MRI brain (abscess or encephalitis) Blood cultures
	Brain Tumor	Seizures may be the first presentation of a mass lesion. Often focal onset	Persistent headaches, focal deficits, papilledema	Cognitive decline, weight loss	MRI brain with contrast (to identify lesions)
	Neurodegenerative causes	Longstanding history of cognitive decline Often focal though may be generalised	Cognitive impairment, progressive neurodegenerative signs	Parkinsons/ Huntington's-motor symptoms Behavioural changes	Investigate for other causes of the seizure
Cardiovascular Causes	Cardiac Arrhythmias	Sudden collapse with seizure-like activity due to cerebral hypoperfusion	Normal neurological exam between episodes	Palpitations, syncope, family history of sudden cardiac death	ECG ± Holter monitor

	Hypertensive Encephalopathy	Seizures, confusion, and vision changes in the context of severe hypertension	Marked hypertension, papilledema	Headache, vomiting, visual changes	Check blood pressure- SBP >=180 and/or DBP >=120 Fundoscopy (papilledema). CT/MRI brain (white matter changes or edema)
Metabolic and Systemic causes	Hypoglycaemia and hyperglycaemia	Altered consciousness, seizures, confusion	Tachycardia, diaphoresis (hypoglycemia); dehydration in hyperglycemia	History of diabetes or medication errors	Blood glucose levels HbA1c (to assess diabetes control)
	Electrolyte Imbalance	Generalized tonic-clonic seizures with no preceding aura	Often normal exam post-seizure	Muscle cramps, fatigue, confusion	Serum sodium, calcium, magnesium, potassium
	Renal or Hepatic Failure	Seizures due to uremic or hepatic encephalopathy	Asterixis, jaundice, or peripheral oedema	Nausea, pruritus	U&E, creatinine (renal function). LFTs, ammonia levels (hepatic function)
Toxicological causes	Alcohol Withdrawal	Seizures occurring 6–48 hours after last alcohol intake	Tremors, tachycardia, diaphoresis	Tremor, confusion, agitation, psychotic symptoms, fast pulse, sweating, fever	Detailed alcohol history
	Drug-Induced Seizures	Overdose of tricyclic antidepressants, cocaine, amphetamines, etc	Altered mental status, abnormal pupils, or arrhythmias	Hyperthermia, agitation	Toxicology screen. ECG (for conduction abnormalities)
Pregnancy-Related causes	Eclampsia	Seizures occurring >20 weeks gestation or postpartum, often in hypertensive women	Hypertension, proteinuria, edema	Severe headache, visual disturbances	BP monitoring. Urinalysis for proteinuria. Blood tests (LFTs, platelets)
Psychogenic Causes	Non-Epileptic Attack Disorder (NEAD)	Episodes resembling seizures without electrical activity on EEG. Often prolonged with emotional triggers	Normal neurological exam	History of trauma or psychiatric illness	EEG during an event. Psychiatric assessment

TYPES OF SEIZURE

Focal Seizures

- Begin on one side of the brain, affecting awareness, behavior, sensation, or movements (typically on one side of the body).
- Can spread to both sides, causing loss of consciousness and bilateral movements.

Generalized Seizures

- Start on both sides of the brain simultaneously.
- Usually causes loss of consciousness and bilateral abnormal movements.

Describing Seizure Movements

- **Tonic**: Stiffening of muscles.
- **Atonic**: Sudden loss of muscle strength or tone.
- **Myoclonic**: Brief, rapid jerking movements.

Top tip

- Postictal phenomena tender to only occur after generalised tonic and/or clonic seizures
- Do not restrain the patient or put anything in their mouth (they won't swallow their tongue)
- Remember to repeatedly go back and reassess the patient after any intervention
- In children assess for developmental abnormalities or regression.

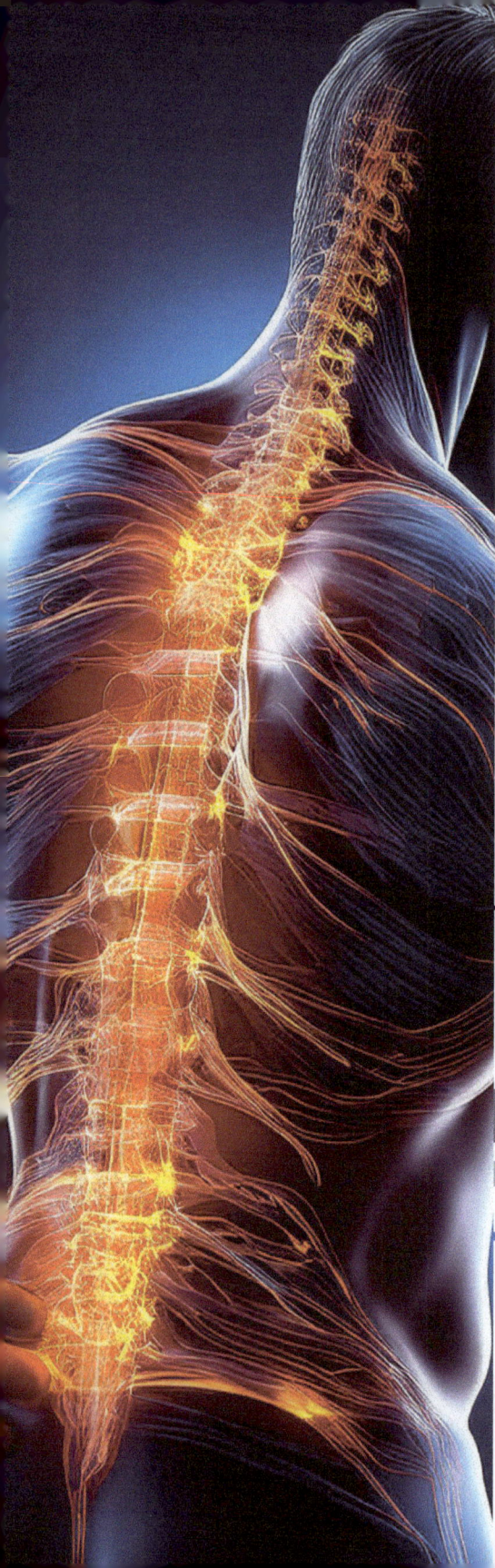

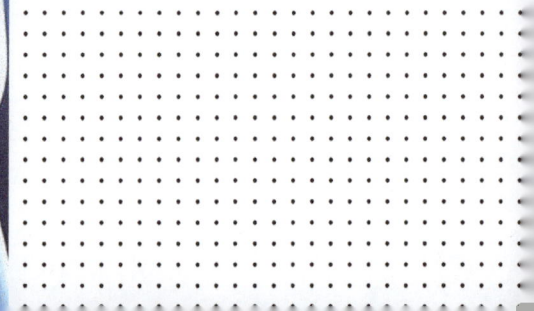

27
Back pain

■ **Back pain** is one of the most common reasons for seeking medical attention, ranging from benign causes like mechanical strain to serious, life-threatening conditions such as spinal cord compression or aortic aneurysm. Accurate diagnosis requires distinguishing between red flag symptoms that suggest serious underlying pathology and benign causes that can be managed conservatively. A systematic history, physical examination, and appropriate investigations form the cornerstone of evaluating and managing back pain effectively.

Diagnostic sieves
■ □ ■ +

Back Pain Red Flags

History

- Constant, unrelenting pain, especially at night
- Pain not exacerbated by movement
- Thoracic pain (associated with malignancy)
- Bladder or bowel dysfunction (incontinence or retention)
- Fever, chills, rigours
- Unexplained weight loss
- Morning stiffness >30 minutes
- Cancer History (Prostate, Renal, Breast, Lung especially)
- Alcohol excess
- IV Drug User
- Immunocompromised

Examination

- Leg weakness
- Saddle anaesthesia (numbness in the groin or perianal area)
- Sensory loss
- Pulsatile abdominal mass
- Severe abdominal or flank pain radiating to the back
- Foot drop
- Arrhythmia

History Taking - Important points

1. SITE:
- Where is the pain located?
- Pain's location helps identify potential causes, such as mechanical issues (lower back), serious conditions like aortic aneurysm (thoracic), or visceral causes like renal colic (flank).

2. ONSET:
- When did the pain start? Was it sudden or gradual?
- Sudden pain may indicate acute conditions like fractures or aortic aneurysm; gradual onset suggests degenerative or inflammatory processes.

3. CHARACTERISTICS:
- How does the pain feel (e.g., sharp, dull, aching, burning)?
- Sharp or burning pain may indicate nerve involvement, while dull or aching pain is more likely mechanical or musculoskeletal.

4. RADIATES:
- Does it radiate to other areas (e.g. legs, groin)?
- Radiating pain to the legs suggests nerve root compression (e.g., sciatica); to the groin could indicate referred pain from the kidneys or pelvis.

5. ASSOCIATED SYMPTOMS:
Numbness, tingling, weakness, or loss of bowel/bladder control?
- Suggests neurological involvement like spinal cord compression or cauda equina syndrome.

Fever, weight loss, night sweats, or fatigue?
- Indicative of systemic or infectious causes like malignancy or osteomyelitis.

Abdominal, chest, or pelvic pain?
- Points to referred pain from visceral conditions like pancreatitis or renal colic.

6. EXACERBATING/RELIEVING FACTORS:
- What makes the pain worse or better (e.g., movement, rest, specific postures)?
- Helps differentiate mechanical pain (worse with movement) from inflammatory pain (better with activity) or systemic causes.

7. TIMING:
- Is the pain constant, intermittent, or worse at a particular time (e.g. night, morning)?
- Night pain raises concerns for malignancy or infection, while morning stiffness suggests inflammatory conditions like ankylosing spondylitis.

8. PAST MEDICAL HISTORY
- Do you have a personal history of cancer?
- Have you ever had any previous issues with your back? Have you had similar episodes in the past?
- Have you had a recent injury or fall?

9. SOCIAL HISTORY
- Mobility: Are you able to walk, bend, or perform daily activities?
- Work/Activity: Has the pain affected your work or hobbies?
- Have you ever injected drugs into yourself?

Are you missing something?

SPINAL CORD COMPRESSION
- Presents with progressive neurological symptoms such as leg weakness, saddle anesthesia, or bowel/bladder dysfunction.
- Common causes include disc herniation, tumors (e.g., metastatic cancer), or epidural abscesses.
- Urgent MRI is critical for diagnosis, as delayed treatment may lead to permanent neurological damage.
- Management typically involves urgent surgical decompression or radiotherapy for malignancy-associated compression.

Diagnostic sieves
■ ■ ■ +

Serious diagnoses to consider

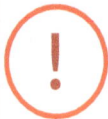

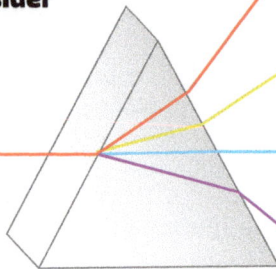

Spinal Cord Compression

Infections:
- Epidural Abscess,
- Osteomyelitis,
- Discitis.

Malignancy

Aortic Aneurysm

! SERIOUS SYMPTOMS!

- Saddle anesthesia: Indicates **cauda equina syndrome**, a medical emergency requiring immediate intervention.
- Leg weakness or foot drop: Suggests **nerve root compression, spinal cord compression,** or **severe lumbar radiculopathy.**
- Pulsatile abdominal mass: Associated with **abdominal aortic aneurysm (AAA)**, particularly concerning if coupled with back or abdominal pain.
- Severe unrelenting pain at night: Raises concerns for **malignancy** (e.g., spinal metastases) or **infection** (e.g., osteomyelitis, discitis).
- Fever, chills, or systemic symptoms: Points to infectious causes like **epidural abscess, discitis, or systemic infections**

! SERIOUS SIGNS!

- Unexplained weight loss: Suggests **malignancy** (e.g., multiple myeloma, metastases) or **systemic infection.**
- Morning stiffness >30 minutes: Indicative of **inflammatory conditions like ankylosing spondylitis or other spondyloarthropathies.**
- Pain radiating to the groin or legs: Suggests **nerve root irritation** (e.g., herniated disc, lumbar radiculopathy) or **referred pain from renal or pelvic pathology.**
- Severe pain unresponsive to movement or rest: Suggestive of **spinal metastases, severe infection, or advanced inflammatory conditions.**

Differential diagnoses using the VITAMIN-C acronym

Category	Differential Diagnosis
V - Vascular	Aortic aneurysm
I - Infectious	Epidural abscess, discitis, pyelonephritis
T - Trauma	Vertebral fractures
A - Autoimmune	Ankylosing spondylitis, sacroiliitis
M - Metabolic	Osteoporosis, Paget's disease, osteomalacia
I - Idiopathic/Functional	Mechanical back pain
N - Neoplastic	Spinal metastases, multiple myeloma
C - Congenital	Spondylolysis, scoliosis

INFECTION OF THE SPINE

- Includes conditions like discitis, osteomyelitis, and epidural abscess.
- Symptoms often feature localized back pain, fever, and systemic signs like chills or weight loss.
- Risk factors include IV drug use, immunosuppression, or recent spinal procedures.
- Diagnosis requires MRI with contrast, blood cultures, and inflammatory markers (e.g., CRP, ESR).
- Treatment involves long-term antibiotics and surgical drainage if abscesses or instability are present.

AORTIC ANEURYSM

- Characterized by severe, sudden back or abdominal pain, often described as "tearing" or "ripping."
- Risk factors include hypertension, smoking, atherosclerosis, and connective tissue disorders like Marfan syndrome.
- A pulsatile abdominal mass may be palpable, and rupture can cause hypotension and shock.
- Imaging with CT angiography or bedside ultrasound confirms the diagnosis.
- Treatment involves urgent surgical repair for rupture or endovascular aneurysm repair (EVAR) for elective cases.
- Always consider cauda equina syndrome in patients with saddle anesthesia, bowel or bladder dysfunction, and severe leg weakness.
- Suspect spinal infection (e.g., epidural abscess) in patients with fever, localized back pain, and risk factors like IV drug use or immunosuppression.
- Aortic aneurysm rupture requires urgent diagnosis if severe, sudden back or abdominal pain is associated with hypotension or a pulsatile mass.

Top Tips

- MRI for nerve or spinal cord pathology, CT for vascular issues.

Spinal Examination Summary:

- Inspect posture, gait, deformities, and systemic signs; palpate spine and joints for tenderness or deformities;
- Assess lumbar range of motion and pain; perform neurological exam (motor strength, reflexes, sensation, SLR, femoral stretch test);
- Conduct special tests (e.g., Schober's test for mobility); and include systemic examination for referred pain causes.

Straight leg raise (SLR): Positive if lifting the leg causes radicular pain below the knee, suggesting nerve root irritation
https://www.aliem.com/trick-of-trade-crossed-straight-leg/

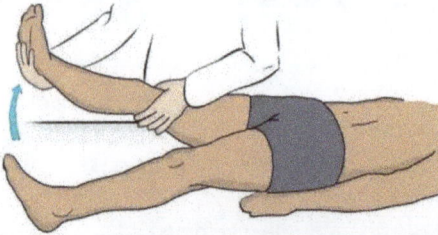

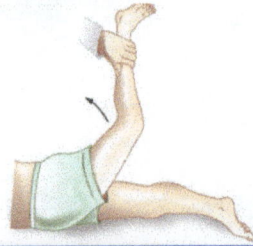

Femoral nerve stretch test: Assess for pain in the anterior thigh for higher nerve root involvement (L2-L4).
www.aliem.com/trick-of-trade-crossed-straight-leg/

Bone profile considerations in back pain assessment

Bone disease	Calcium	Phosphate	ALP	Additional blood tests
Osteoporosis	Normal	Normal	Normal	-
Osteomalacia	Low	Low	High	-
Pagets	Normal	Normal	Very high	-
Myeloma	High	Normal-High	Normal	Deranged renal function
Bone metastasis	High	Normal-High	High	-
Primary hyperparathyroidism	High	Low-Normal	Normal-High	High PTH

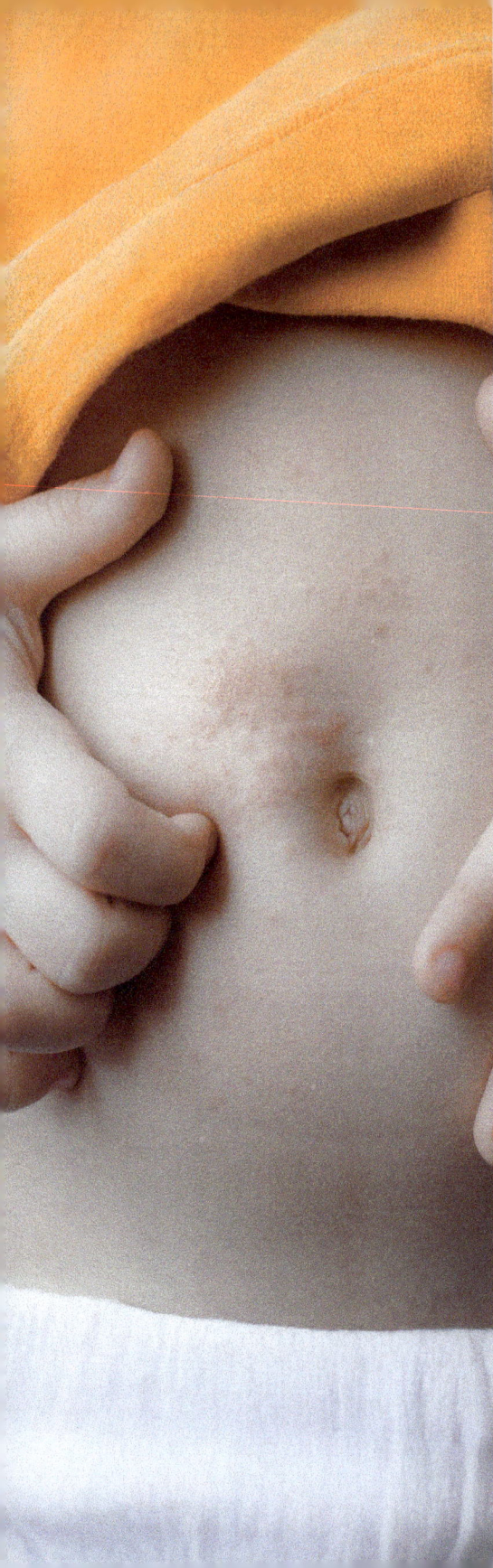

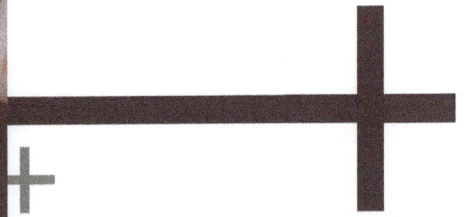

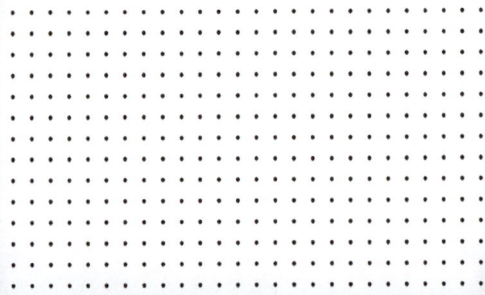

28

Rash

Rashes are common presentations in medical practice, ranging from benign self-limiting conditions to life-threatening systemic diseases. Recognizing key features and red flags is critical to identifying serious causes that require urgent intervention. A systematic approach that includes history taking, examination, and relevant investigations is essential for accurate diagnosis and management.

Diagnostic sieves

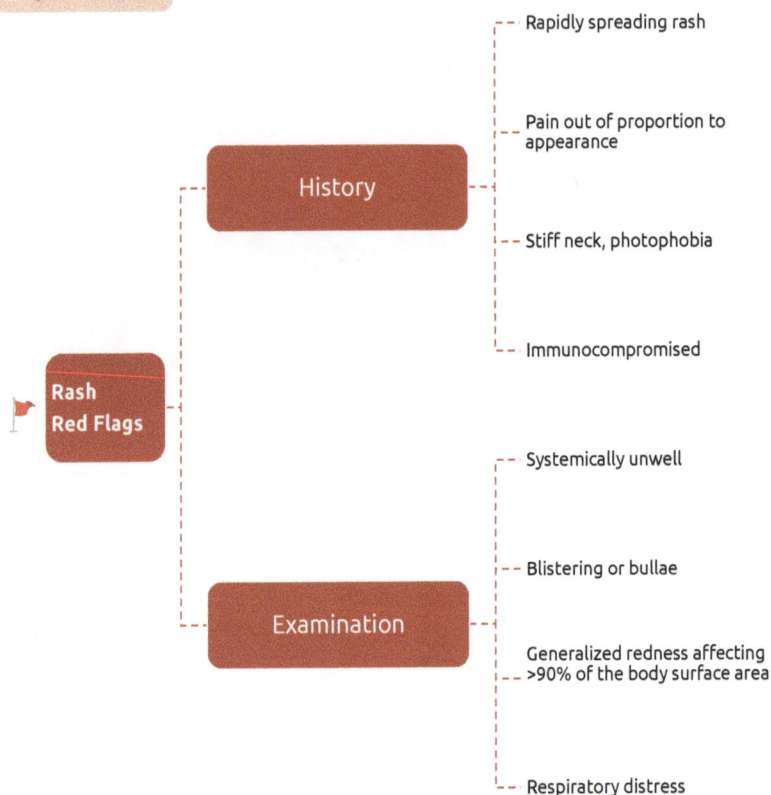

Rash Red Flags

History
- Rapidly spreading rash
- Pain out of proportion to appearance
- Stiff neck, photophobia
- Immunocompromised

Examination
- Systemically unwell
- Blistering or bullae
- Generalized redness affecting >90% of the body surface area
- Respiratory distress

⚠ SERIOUS DIAGNOSES!

- Meningococcal sepsis
- Toxic shock syndrome
- Necrotising fasciitis
- Staphylococcal scalded skin syndrome
- Herpes zoster (disseminated or ocular)
- Rash in immunocompromised individuals
- Pemphigus vulgaris, Bullous pemphigoid
- Syphilis (secondary or tertiary)
- Disseminated gonococcal infection
- Endocarditis with septic emboli
- Stevens-Johnson Syndrome (SJS)
- Toxic Epidermal Necrolysis (TEN)
- Drug Reaction with Eosinophilia and Systemic Symptoms (DRESS)
- Vasculitis (e.g., Henoch-Schönlein Purpura, ANCA-associated vasculitis)
- Systemic lupus erythematosus (SLE)
- Dermatomyositis
- Erythroderma
- Leukemia (e.g. acute leukemia with petechiae)
- Cutaneous T-cell lymphoma (e.g. mycosis fungoides)

History Taking - Important points

I. PRESENTING COMPLAINT

Use the SOCRATES framework to structure the questions:

Site

- "Where did the rash first appear?"
- "Has it spread to other areas of your body?"

Onset

- "When did you first notice the rash?"
- "Was the onset sudden or gradual?"
- "Did anything unusual happen before the rash started (e.g., new medications, travel, illness, or contact with allergens)?"

Character

- "What does the rash look like? Are there blisters, raised areas, or flat spots?"
- "How does it feel? Is it itchy, painful, or tender?"
- "Does it ooze, bleed, or scab over?"
- "How many lesions are there? What shape or pattern do they have?"

Radiation

- "Does the rash or any associated pain spread to other areas?"

Associated Symptoms

- "Do you have any other symptoms, such as fever, chills, joint pain, or weight loss?"
- "Is the rash associated with itching, burning, or tingling?"
- "Have you noticed any swelling, redness, or pus in the affected area?"
- "Are you experiencing fatigue, sore throat, or a general feeling of being unwell?"

Time Course

- "How has the rash changed over time?"
- "Have you ever had a rash like this before?"
- "When you had it previously, how was it treated?"

Exacerbating or Relieving Factors

- "Does anything make the rash better or worse (e.g., heat, cold, scratching, medications)?"

- "Have you tried any home remedies or over-the-counter treatments?"

Severity

- "On a scale of 0-10, how uncomfortable or painful is the rash?"

2. DRUG HISTORY

- "Are you taking any new medications or supplements?"
- "Have you started or stopped any medications recently?"
- "Have you previously reacted to medications?

3. SOCIAL AND ENVIRONMENTAL HISTORY

- "Have you traveled recently or been exposed to new environments?"
- "Do you work with any substances that could irritate the skin (e.g., chemicals, plants)?"
- "Do you have pets or contact with animals?"

4. CONTACT HISTORY

- "Have you been in contact with anyone who has a rash or infectious illness (e.g., chickenpox, measles)?"

5. SYSTEMS REVIEW

Ask specifically about:

- Fever and malaise (suggesting infection or systemic disease)
- Joint pain or swelling (indicative of autoimmune conditions)
- Weight loss (possible malignancy or systemic disease)
- Respiratory symptoms (e.g., cough, wheeze – might suggest drug reactions or vasculitis)

Key Examination

GENERAL INSPECTION

Lesion Distribution:

- Acral: Hands/feet (e.g., hand, foot, and mouth disease).
- Extensor: Elbows/knees (e.g., psoriasis).
- Flexural: Axillae/genital region (e.g., eczema).
- Follicular: Sebaceous-rich areas (e.g., acne).
- Dermatomal: Confined to dermatomes, not crossing midline (e.g., herpes zoster).
- Seborrhoeic: Face/scalp (e.g., seborrhoeic dermatitis).

Objects/Equipment:

- Look for medications, dressings, or aids that indicate underlying conditions.

CLOSE INSPECTION

Size and Configuration:

- Measure the lesions.
- Assess shapes: discrete, confluent, linear, discoid, annular, or target-like.

Colour:

- Erythematous: Red and blanching (e.g., inflammation).
- Purpuric: Reddish-purple, non-blanching (e.g., vasculitis).
- Hyperpigmented: Darker skin areas (e.g., Addison's disease).
- Hypopigmented/Depigmented: Pale or white (e.g., pityriasis versicolor or vitiligo).

Morphology:

- Primary lesions: Macule, patch, papule, plaque, vesicle, pustule, wheal.
- Secondary lesions: Excoriations, crusts, scales, ulcers, scars.

PALPATION

Surface Characteristics:

- Texture: Smooth or rough.
- Elevation: Flat, raised, or depressed.
- Crusts: Determine underlying tissue integrity.
- Temperature: Warmth suggests infection/inflammation.

Deeper Characteristics:

- Consistency: Hard, firm, or soft.
- Fluctuance: Indicates fluid-filled lesions (e.g., abscess).
- Mobility: Fixed or mobile.
- Tenderness: Suggests inflammation or infection.

SYSTEMIC EXAMINATION

Hands and Nails:

- Nail changes: Pitting (eczema, psoriasis), onycholysis (psoriasis, fungal infections), koilonychia (anaemia).
- Hand and fingers: Osler nodes/Janeway lesions

Elbows:

- Look for psoriasis plaques, rheumatoid nodules, or xanthomas.

Hair and Scalp:

- Hair loss: Alopecia areata (patchy), alopecia totalis (scalp-wide).
- Excess growth: Hirsutism (androgenic), hypertrichosis (non-androgenic).
- Scalp lesions: Psoriasis (scaly plaques), seborrhoeic dermatitis (diffuse scaling).

Mucous Membranes:

- Inspect for bullae (e.g., bullous pemphigoid), Wickham's striae (lichen planus), or hyperpigmented macules (Peutz-Jeghers syndrome).

5. SPECIFIC ASSESSMENT FOR PIGMENTED LESIONS

- Use ABCDE criteria:
- Asymmetry
- Border irregularity
- Colour variation
- Diameter
- Elevation/Evolution

Differential diagnosis

MENINGOCOCCAL SEPSIS

Rash Type: Non-Blanching (Purpuric/Petechial) Rash

Key Features:

- Rapid onset of fever, vomiting, and headache.
- Purpuric/petechial rash, often starting on the extremities and spreading centrally.
- Symptoms of sepsis (e.g., hypotension, tachycardia).
- Possible meningitis symptoms (e.g., neck stiffness, photophobia).

Associated Symptoms:

- Fever, hypotension, cold extremities, altered consciousness.

Examination Findings:

- Non-blanching petechiae, purpura.
- Shock (low blood pressure, high heart rate).
- Meningism (neck stiffness, Kernig's/ Brudzinski signs).

Investigations:

- Blood cultures, throat swab.
- PCR for Neisseria meningitidis.
- Full blood count (FBC) for leukocytosis.
- Coagulation studies (e.g., D-dimer).
- Serum lactate for sepsis.

TOXIC SHOCK SYNDROME (TSS)

Rash Type: Erythematous (Blanching) Rash

Key Features:

- Fever >38.9°C, hypotension, multi-organ involvement.
- Diffuse maculopapular rash, which may evolve into desquamation.
- Rapid onset of symptoms.

Associated Symptoms:

- Fever, hypotension, multisystem involvement (renal, hepatic, cardiac, GI).

Examination Findings:

- Red, blanching maculopapular rash.
- Desquamation (peeling skin) 1-2 weeks after rash onset.
- Shock, altered mental status.

Investigations:

- Blood cultures (e.g., Staphylococcus aureus, Streptococcus pyogenes).
- Tissue cultures from suspected sites (e.g., nasal or throat swabs).
- Serum electrolytes and renal function tests.
- Full blood count (FBC) and liver function tests (LFTs).
- Coagulation profile (e.g., PT, aPTT).
-

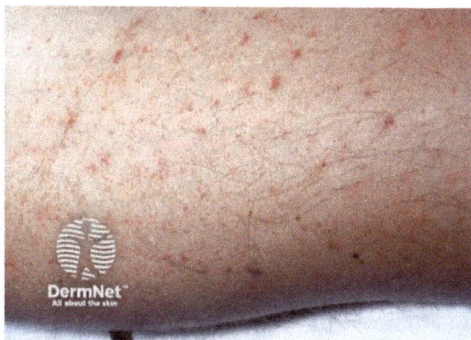

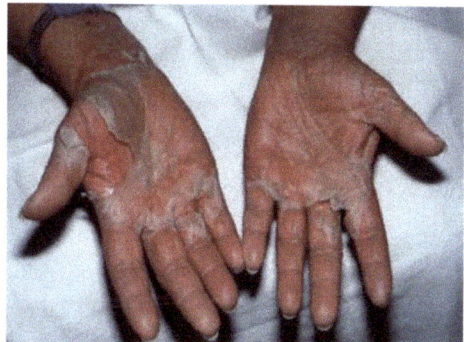

Figure 28.1
Meningococcal rash (left); courtesy dermnetnz.org
Toxic Shock desquamating rash (right); courtesy rmi.edu.pk/disease/toxic-shock-syndrome

NECROTIZING FASCIITIS

Rash Type: Erythematous (Blanching) Rash

Key Features:

- Rapid progression of pain, often following trauma or surgery.
- Erythema, swelling, and tenderness at the site of infection.
- Systemic signs of infection (fever, shock).

Associated Symptoms:

- Severe pain disproportionate to the physical findings, fever, chills.

Examination Findings:

- Red, swollen, warm skin over the affected area.
- Crepitus or gas production (in gas gangrene).
- Systemic signs of sepsis (tachycardia, hypotension).

Investigations:

- CT or MRI to assess the extent of tissue involvement.
- Blood cultures.
- Tissue biopsy or aspirate for microbiological analysis.
- FBC for leukocytosis.
- Lactate levels to assess sepsis.

HERPES ZOSTER (DISSEMINATED OR INVOLVING CRITICAL AREAS)

Rash Type: Vesicular or Bullous Rash

Key Features:

- Vesicular rash in a dermatomal distribution.
- Severe pain (post-herpetic neuralgia in some cases).
- Can affect the eye (herpes zoster ophthalmicus).

Associated Symptoms:

- Burning, tingling, or itching in the affected area before the rash appears.
- Fever, malaise, and fatigue.

Examination Findings:

- Vesicles on an erythematous base.
- If ophthalmic involvement: conjunctivitis, corneal lesions.

Investigations:

- PCR or direct fluorescent antibody testing from skin lesion.
- Blood test for varicella zoster virus (VZV) antibodies.
- Eye exam if the eye is involved (slit-lamp examination).

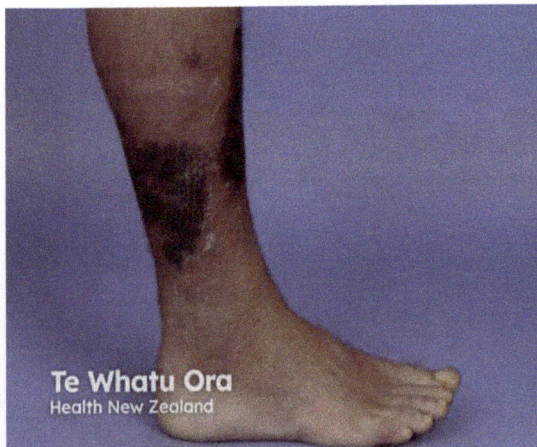

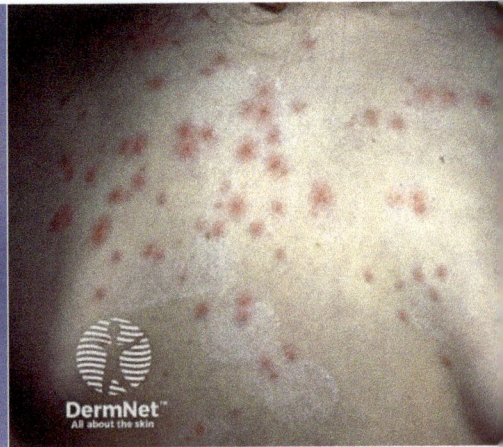

Te Whatu Ora
Health New Zealand

DermNet™
All about the skin

Figure 28.2
Necrotizing fascitis (left); courtesy dermnetnz.org/topics/necrotising-fasciitis
Chicken pox (Varicella zoster) (right); courtesy dermnetnz.org/topics/varicella-images

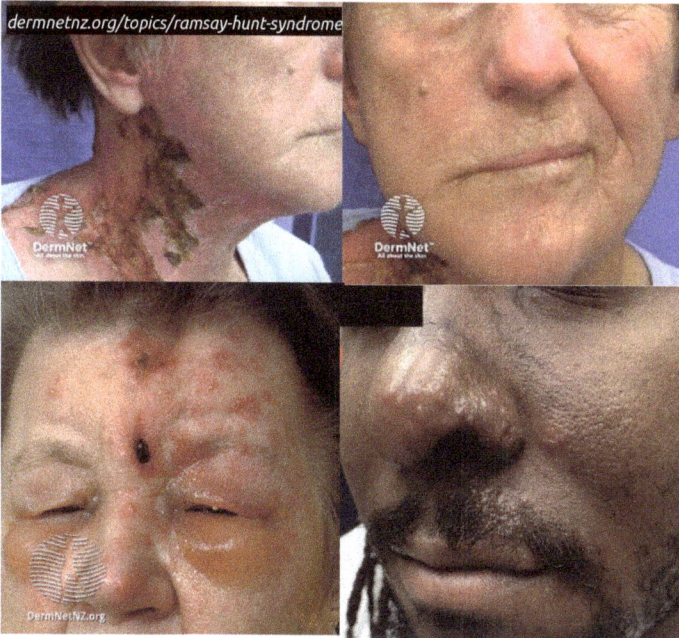

Figure 28.3
Top left & right:
Ramsay-Hunt Syndrome

Bottom left:
Herpes zoster
opthalmicus

Bottom right:
Hutchinsons sign

dermnetnz.org/imagedetail/12146-eyelid-herpes-zoster-ophthalmicus
jetem.org/hutchinsons_sign

PEMPHIGUS VULGARIS

Rash Type: Vesicular or Bullous Rash

Key Features:

- Flaccid blisters that rupture easily, leaving painful erosions.
- Nikolsky sign positive.
- Autoimmune disease due to desmoglein antibodies.

Associated Symptoms:

- Oral mucosal involvement (painful sores).
- Fever, malaise.

Examination Findings:

- Flaccid bullae, erosions, ulcerations.
- Positive Nikolsky sign.

Investigations:

- Skin biopsy for histopathology (Acantholysis).
- Direct immunofluorescence for intercellular IgG deposits.
- Serum anti-desmoglein antibodies.

BULLOUS PEMPHIGOID

Rash Type: Vesicular or Bullous Rash

Key Features:

- Tense, large bullae on erythematous or normal-appearing skin.
- Predominantly in elderly individuals.
- Autoimmune condition involving antibodies against basement membrane.

Associated Symptoms:

- Itching (pruritus).
- Rare systemic involvement.

Examination Findings:

- Tense bullae, often on lower abdomen or flexural areas.
- Negative Nikolsky sign.

Investigations:

- Skin biopsy with direct immunofluorescence for C3 and IgG.
- Serum testing for anti-BP180 and anti-BP230 antibodies.

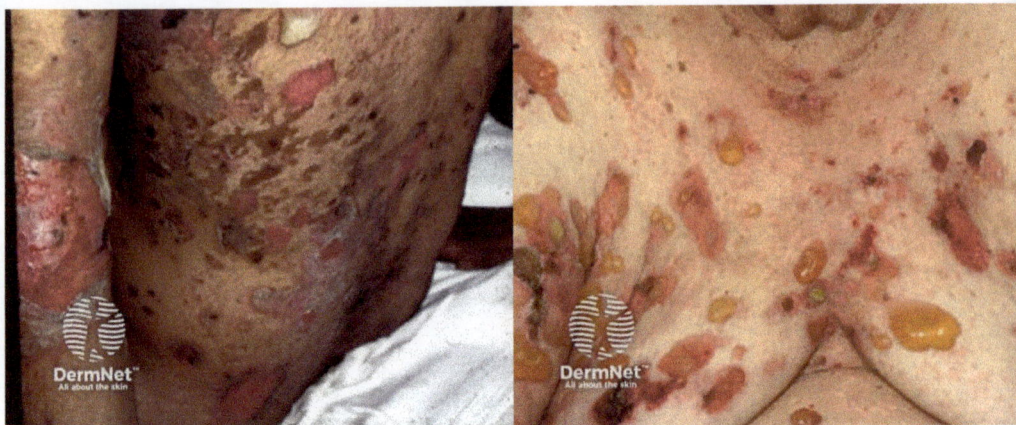

Figure 28.4: Pemphigus vulgaris (left); courtesy dermnetnz.org/topics/pemphigus-vulgaris
Bullous pemphigoid (right); courtesy dermnetnz.org/topics/bullous-pemphigoid
Figure 28.5: SJS/TEN (bottom);
Courtesy https://coreem.net/podcast/episode-162-0-stevens-johnson-syndrome-toxic-epidermal-necrolysis/

Stevens-Johnson Syndrome (SJS)/Toxic Epidermal Necrolysis (TEN)

The rash in SJS/TEN consists of painful pink to dark-red spots that may blister and usually involves the skin, lips, mouth, eyes, and genitals.

Early-stage rash

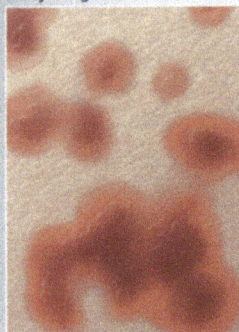

Flat or slightly raised pink spots with dark-red centers

Middle-stage rash

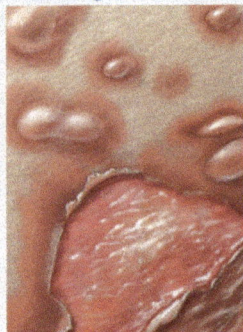

Blistering, peeling skin

Typical rash distribution

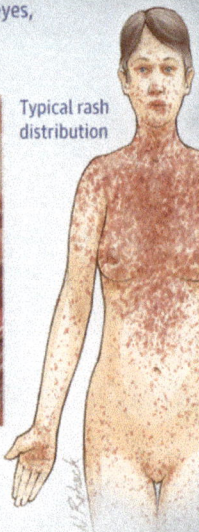

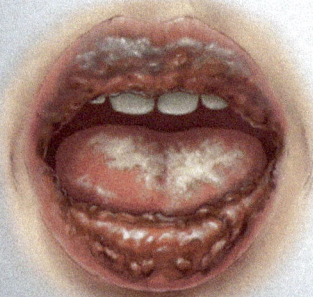

Redness, blisters, and erosions of the lips and inside of the mouth

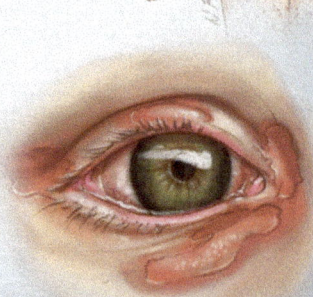

Redness, irritation, pain, and erosions of the eyelids and eye

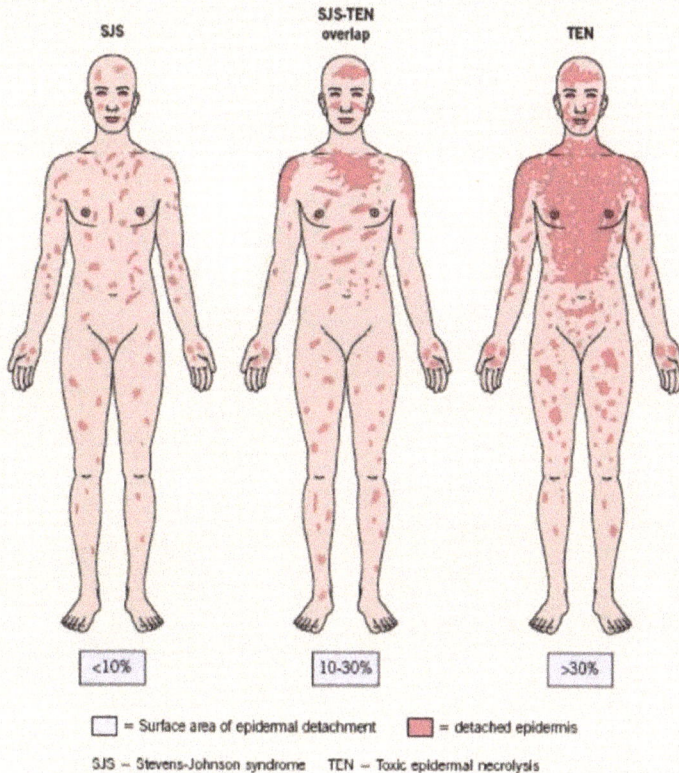

SJS   SJS-TEN   TEN
             overlap

<10%   10-30%   >30%

☐ = Surface area of epidermal detachment   ▨ = detached epidermis

SJS – Stevens-Johnson syndrome   TEN – Toxic epidermal necrolysis

Figure 28.6: SJS - TENS distribution
Courtesy: ojrd.biomedcentral.com/articles/10.1186/1750-1172-5-39

STEVENS-JOHNSON SYNDROME (SJS)/ TOXIC EPIDERMAL NECROLYSIS (TEN)

Rash Type: Vesicular or Bullous Rash

SJS <10% of body surface, TEN >30% of body surface, 10-30% SJS-TEN overlap

Key Features:

- Severe mucosal involvement (oral, ocular, genital).
- Target lesions or erythematous plaques that progress to blistering.
- Usually triggered by medications or infections.
- Extensive, widespread epidermal detachment, often affecting large areas of the body.

Associated Symptoms:

- Fever, malaise, conjunctivitis, and/or urethritis.
- Mucosal involvement (oral, genital, ocular)

Examination Findings:

- Large bullae, widespread erythema, & detachment of the epidermis (positive Nikolsky's sign).
- Mucosal lesions (oral ulcers, conjunctivitis).
- Severe dehydration & electrolyte imbalances.

Investigations:

- Skin biopsy for histopathology.
- Blood tests to assess the severity (FBC, liver, kidney function).
- Identify any precipitating drugs (e.g., anticonvulsants, antibiotics).
- Skin cultures to rule out secondary infection.
- Electrolyte monitoring and renal function tests

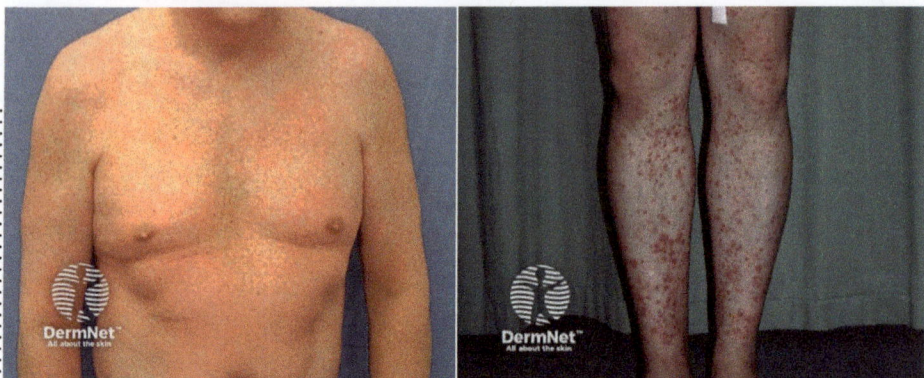

Figure 28.7: Drug hypersensitivity syndrome (left); *Courtesy: dermnetnz.org/topics/drug-hypersensitivity-syndrome*
Henoch Schonlein purpura (right); *Courtesy: dermnetnz.org/topics/vasculitis-images*

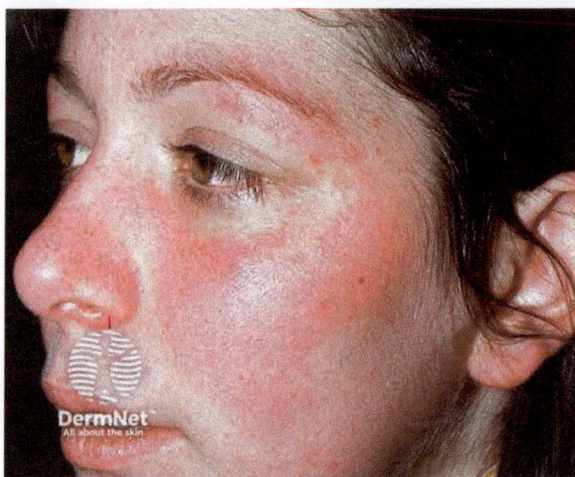

Figure 28.8: Systemic lupus Erythematosus (above);
courtesy: dermnetnz.org/topics/systemic-lupus-erythematosus

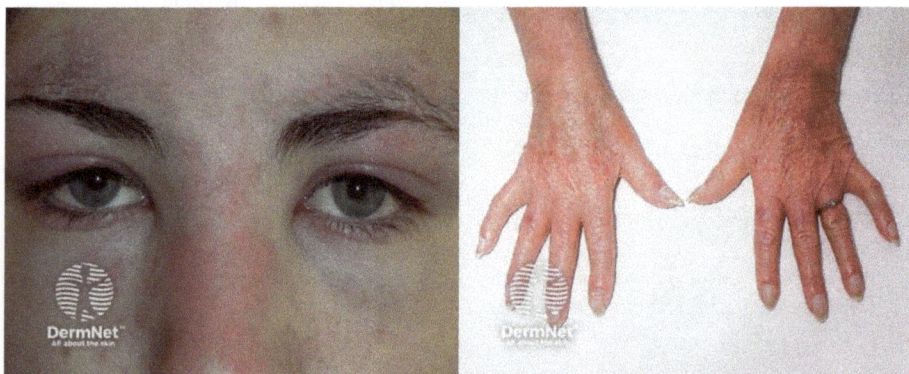

Figure 28.9 Heliotrope rash (left); Gottrons papules (right). Both indicate Dermatomyositis
courtesy: dermnetnz.org/topics/dermatomyositis-images

DRUG REACTION WITH EOSINOPHILIA AND SYSTEMIC SYMPTOMS (DRESS)

Rash Type: Maculopapular Rash

Key Features:

- Fever, eosinophilia, and a rash often starting on the trunk.
- History of recent drug exposure (e.g., anticonvulsants, sulfonamides).
- Multi-organ involvement (liver, kidneys, lungs).

Associated Symptoms:

- Fever, facial edema, lymphadenopathy, and sore throat.
- Hepatitis, renal dysfunction, pneumonitis.

Examination Findings:

- Morbilliform maculopapular rash, often with facial swelling.
- Lymphadenopathy, hepatomegaly, or splenomegaly.

Investigations:

- Blood tests for eosinophilia.
- Liver and kidney function tests (ALT, AST, creatinine, BUN).
- Skin biopsy for histopathological evaluation.
- Discontinuation of suspected drug and supportive care.

VASCULITIS (E.G., HENOCH-SCHÖNLEIN PURPURA, ANCA-ASSOCIATED VASCULITIS)

Rash Type: Non-Blanching (Purpuric/Petechial) Rash

Key Features:

- Henoch-Schönlein purpura (HSP) typically presents with purpura over the lower extremities and buttocks.
- Systemic vasculitis involving the skin, joints, kidneys, and GI tract.
- ANCA-associated vasculitis (e.g., granulomatosis with polyangiitis) often has pulmonary and renal involvement.

Associated Symptoms:

- Joint pain (in HSP), abdominal pain (GI involvement in HSP).
- Renal involvement (hematuria, proteinuria), respiratory symptoms in ANCA vasculitis.

Examination Findings:

- Non-blanching purpura on the lower limbs in HSP.
- Nodules or ulcerations in the oral cavity or respiratory tract (in ANCA-associated vasculitis).
- Abdominal tenderness or signs of GI hemorrhage.

Investigations:

- FBC, renal function tests, urinalysis (e.g., hematuria).
- ANCA testing for ANCA-associated vasculitis.
- Skin biopsy for histopathology to assess the vasculitis type.
- Abdominal ultrasound (for HSP-related GI involvement)

SYSTEMIC LUPUS ERYTHEMATOSUS (SLE)

Rash Type: Maculopapular Rash or Scaly or Plaque-Like Rash

Key Features:

- Classic butterfly-shaped malar rash over the nose and cheeks.
- Photosensitivity exacerbating the rash.
- Associated with systemic involvement (e.g., renal, neurological).

Associated Symptoms:

- Joint pain, photosensitivity, fatigue.
- Kidney disease (e.g., lupus nephritis), pleuritis.

Examination Findings:

- Butterfly-shaped malar rash, spares the nasolabial folds.
- Discoid lupus (scaly plaques) on sun-exposed areas.
- Oral ulcers, alopecia.

Investigations:

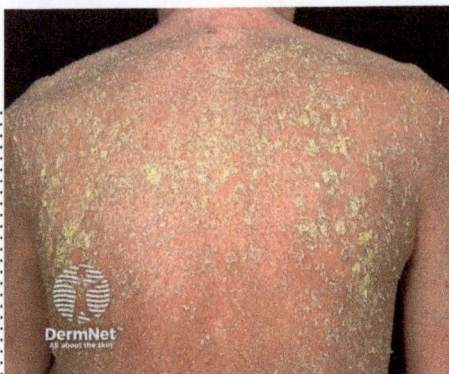

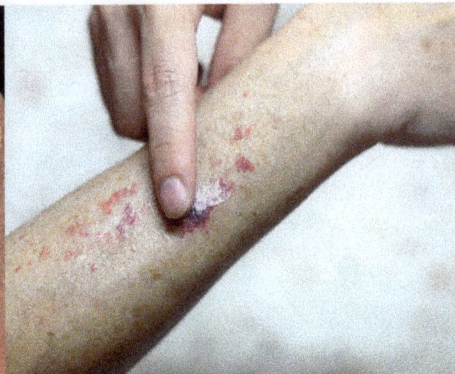

Figure 28.10: Erythroderma (left); Gottrons papules (right). Both indicate Dermatomyositis
dermnetnz.org/topics/erythroderma

Left: Erythroderma; Right: Gottrons papules. Both indicate Dermatomyositis
moffitt.org/cancers/leukemia/faqs/what-do-leukemia-spots-look-like/

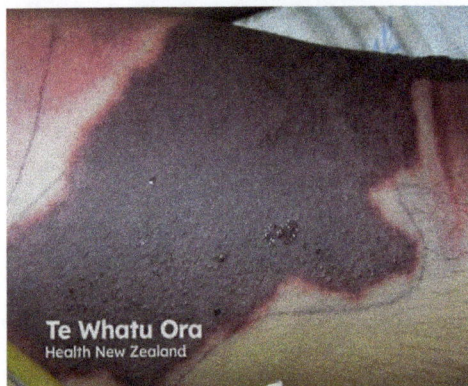

Figure 28.11: Disseminated Intravascular Coagulation
courtesy: dermnetnz.org/topics/disseminated-intravascular-coagulation

- Antinuclear antibody (ANA) testing.
- Anti-dsDNA and anti-Smith antibodies (specific for lupus).
- Complement levels (low C3, C4 in active disease).
- Urinalysis for proteinuria, hematuria.

DERMATOMYOSITIS

Rash Type: Erythematous (Blanching) Rash or Nodular or Papular Rash

Key Features:

- Bilateral, symmetrical erythematous rash over the knuckles (Gottron's papules).
- Heliotrope rash around the eyes.
- Associated muscle weakness.

Associated Symptoms:

- Proximal muscle weakness, dysphagia, respiratory weakness.
- Interstitial lung disease in some cases.

Examination Findings:

- Gottron's papules (erythematous knuckle lesions).
- Heliotrope rash (purple discoloration around the eyes).
- Muscle tenderness and weakness.

Investigations:

- Elevated creatine kinase (CK) levels.
- Muscle biopsy to confirm inflammation.
- Anti-Jo-1 antibodies for a characteristic myositis marker.
- EMG (electromyography) to assess muscle

function.

ERYTHRODERMA

Rash Type: Erythroderma

Key Features:

- Widespread erythema, scaling, and exfoliation affecting >90% of body surface area.
- Often associated with underlying dermatological diseases (e.g., psoriasis, eczema) or systemic disease.

Associated Symptoms:

- Fever, chills, dehydration, hypotension.
- Risk of secondary infections due to skin barrier loss.

Examination Findings:

- Diffuse erythema, scaling, and peeling of the skin.
- Tender, inflamed skin with possible systemic signs of infection.

Investigations:

- Skin biopsy for histopathological evaluation.
- FBC, liver, and kidney function tests.
- Blood cultures if infection is suspected.

LEUKEMIA (E.G., ACUTE LEUKEMIA WITH PETECHIAE)

Rash Type: Non-Blanching (Purpuric/Petechial) Rash

Key Features:

- Petechiae and purpura often seen due to thrombocytopenia.
- Associated with fever, malaise, and lymphadenopathy.
- Leukemia may present with bone pain, splenomegaly, and hepatomegaly.

Associated Symptoms:

- Fatigue, weight loss, recurrent infections
- Bone pain, bleeding tendencies.
- Examination Findings:
- Purpura, petechiae, or bruising.
- Pale skin, hepatosplenomegaly,

lymphadenopathy.

Investigations:

- Blood counts (CBC with peripheral smear showing blasts).
- Bone marrow biopsy to diagnose leukemia.
- Coagulation profile to assess bleeding risk

DISSEMINATED INTRAVASCULAR COAGULATION (DIC)

Rash Type: Non-Blanching (Purpuric/Petechial) Rash or Bruising

Key Features & History:

History:

- Triggering events: sepsis, trauma, malignancy (e.g., leukemia), obstetric complications (e.g., abruptio placentae, amniotic fluid embolism), or severe infections.
- History of prolonged bleeding, bruising, or symptoms of the underlying cause.
- Sudden onset of symptoms in acute DIC or slow progression in chronic cases.

Key Findings:

- Purpura: Widespread non-blanching rash.
- Ecchymoses: Larger areas of bruising.
- Petechiae: Small pinpoint non-blanching spots on the skin or mucous membranes.
- Signs of microvascular thrombosis: cyanosis or ischemia in severe cases.
- Bleeding from multiple sites, e.g., gums, venipuncture sites, or gastrointestinal tract.

Associated Symptoms:

- Symptoms of the underlying condition (e.g., fever in sepsis, abdominal pain in obstetric complications).
- Fatigue, dyspnea, or confusion due to anemia or hypoxia.
- Signs of organ dysfunction due to microthrombi: oliguria (renal impairment), jaundice (liver dysfunction), or altered mental status (neurological involvement).

Investigations:

- Coagulation Profile:

- Prolonged prothrombin time (PT) and activated partial thromboplastin time (aPTT).
- Reduced fibrinogen levels.
- Elevated D-dimer (indicating fibrinolysis).
- Full Blood Count (FBC):
- Thrombocytopenia (reduced platelets).
- Presence of fragmented red blood cells (schistocytes) on peripheral blood smear (microangiopathic hemolysis).

- Fibrin Degradation Products (FDPs): Elevated.
- Organ Function Tests: Assess for liver, kidney, and other systemic dysfunction.
- Underlying Cause Investigations: Blood cultures (sepsis), imaging (malignancy), or obstetric assessments (ultrasound).

www.ingramcontent.com/pod-product-compliance
Lightning Source LLC
Chambersburg PA
CBHW040850210326
41597CB00029B/4789